HYPOMETABOLISM

HYPOMETABOLISM

A CLINICAL STUDY OF 308 CONSECUTIVE CASES

BY

ESBEN KIRK, M. D.

Chief Physician, Medical Department, Holstebro District Hospital, Holstebro, Denmark.

AND

SVEN ANCHER KVORNING, M. D.

Assistant, Pharmacological Department, University of Copenhagen; Former Resident Physician, Medical Department, Holstebro District Hospital, Holstebro, Denmark.

EINAR MUNKSGAARD
PUBLISHER
COPENHAGEN 1946

HEINEMANN
MEDICAL BOOKS-LTD.
LONDON 1946

Translated by
Miss Annie I. Fausbøll, M. A.,
and the Authors.

Printed in Denmark
by
H. P. Hansens Bogtr., Copenhagen

CONTENTS

PREFACE

The present investigation was carried out for the purpose of establishing the frequency of the various forms of hypometabolism, encountered in a medical department, and the symptomatology of these forms.

The study is based on observations made on a large number of patients who were examined shortly after the opening of a medical service in a district of Denmark previously deprived of easy access to specialists in internal medicine. By these examinations a reduction in the metabolic rate was demonstrated in so many instances that a closer investigation of this problem appeared desirable. Besides illustrating the clinical aspects of hypometabolism the results obtained allowed to draw certain conclusions regarding the pathogenesis of the reduced metabolic rate as well as concerning the possibility and advisability of treating the hypometabolism and the disorders which cause it, for which reason it was considered advisable to present this comprehensive material in the form of a monograph.

In order to facilitate the presentation the accompanying text is deliberaty limited, and a review of the previous literature is omitted, concerning which the reader is referred to the extensive surveys in the references.

For valuable advice, especially in the systematic division of the patients in subgroups, we are indebted to Professor Eggert Møller, M. D., University of Copenhagen.

In the numerical treatment of the material various statistical calculations have been carried out by Henry Fibiger Holm, Secretary of the Municipal Statistical Department, Copenhagen.

1. INTRODUCTION

The investigation comprises a clinical study of 308 cases of hypometabolism admitted to the Medical Department of the Holstebro District Hospital during the years 1940, 1941, and 1942. This period corresponds to the first three calendar years of the department's activity. The medical department serves a district in Northwestern Jutland including the cities of Holstebro and Struer and the surrounding counties (see Fig. 1). The population of the two cities is 13.500 and 6.800 respectively, of the rural districts approximately 50.000.

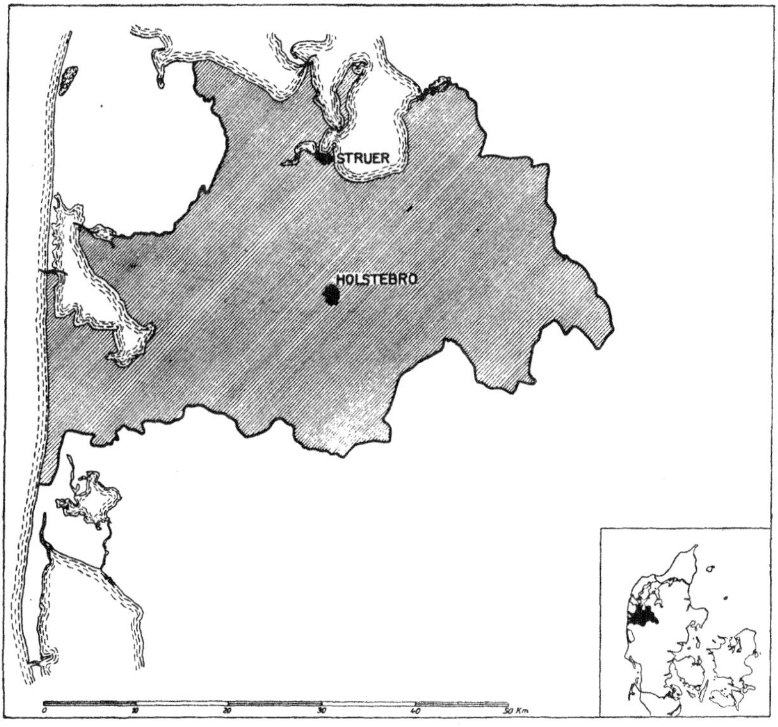

FIG. 1
Map of district served by the Medical Department of the Holstebro District Hospital.

The requirement for including the patients in the hypometabolism group was that the basal metabolism, generally on the basis of a series of determinations, was found to be reduced to 88 p.c. or less. In the period from February 1, 1941 to January 31, 1942, the determination was made on all adult patients whose condition permitted such an examination. In the remaining part of the period (January 1, 1940 to January 31, 1941 and February 1, 1942 to December 31, 1942) the metabolism determinations were not performed on all the admitted patients; the measurements were however employed to such an extent that the majority of patients with hypometabolism from these years must be supposed to be included in the study. The clinical diagnosis was based partly on thorough examinations during the first hospitalisation, partly on, as a rule repeated, post-examinations during subsequent admissions. In numerous cases it was possible to extend these post-examinations to the years 1943, 1944, and 1945, so that for a great number of the patients the observation period was extended to 3—5 years.

For comparison with the hypometabolism group a control material of 190 patients was obtained in the period February 1, 1941 to January 31, 1942. This control group consisted of patients whose metabolism was found to be higher than 88 p.c., who were not feverish, and who did not present symptoms of thyrotoxicosis, diabetes, renal diseases, severe blood diseases, cardiac decompensation or pulmonary insufficiency. From this control group were also excluded some patients whose condition did not permit a determination of their metabolism. Both the patients with hypometabolism and the patients of the control group were subjected to a uniform clinical examination as a supplement to the usual examination of the Department for the purpose of making the observations more easily accessible for comparison and statistic treatment. The data from the case history and the clinical observations for the individual patients with hypometabolism have been entered in the appended tables (Tables I—XIII).

2. OUTLINE OF THE CLINICAL EXAMINATION OF THE PATIENTS

In the above-mentioned supplementary uniform clinical examination of the patients, weight was attached to the following 11 symptoms in the history: chilliness, decreased sweating, fatigue, impairment of memory or reduced power of inculcation, somnolence, depression, dyspepsia, constipation, oliguria, conditions of menstruation, and rheumatism (cf. Table 2). In this connection it should be stated that the term "fatigue" comprises both physical and mental fatigue, since as a rule it was not considered possible to make the patients distinguish between these two forms. For the same reason the symptoms "impaired memory" and "reduced power of inculcation" have been entered in the same column. The term "dyspepsia" comprises both gastric and intestinal complaints, the symptom "rheumatism" both pains in the joints and pains localised to the muscles, tendons, fasciae, and subcutaneous tissues. The information given concerning oliguria must be supposed to be rather uncertain, as these particulars are probably to a greater extent than the others affected by the subjective judgment of the patients and their sense of decorum.

In accordance with the generally accepted view, the authors have regarded certain changes in the skin of the face as characteristic of genuine myxedema. These changes consist in coarse features, a mask-like expression, and puffiness of the eyelids. There is an often marked non-pitting edema with stiff wrinkles of the forehead (see Fig. 2); the skin of the face is dry and scaly, usually pale and slightly yellowish. The physical examination and observation of the patients in addition to these changes of the skin comprise the following 12 symptoms and signs, the evaluation of which does not require special mention: apathy, depression, scantiness of the hair of the scalp, scantiness of eyebrows, hoarseness, enlargement of the thyroid gland, sparseness of axillary and of pubic hair, thickening of the skin and the subcutaneous tissues on the extremities, perniosis, subcutaneous infiltrations, and myalgiae. Further, the pulse rate and the temperature were measured twice daily, and the height and weight of the patients ascertained. The observation from several different measurements of a pulse rate below 50, and a body temperature below 36^0, has in the

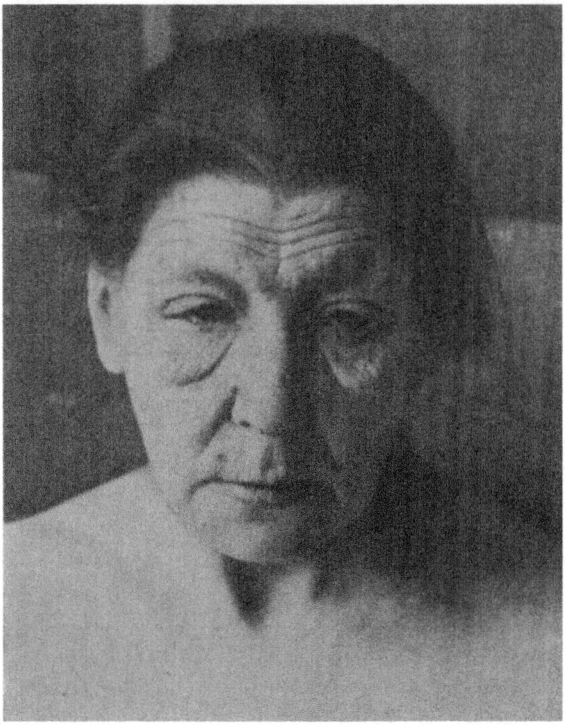

FIG. 2
Photograph of a patient with genuine myxedema.

present exposition been denoted as bradycardia and hypothermia respectively. The calculation of the ideal weight was made according to Broca's formula

$$\text{Ideal weight} = \frac{(\text{Height in centimetres} - 100)}{100} \cdot 90$$

In several cases a measurement of the diuresis was also made and a determination of the serum cholesterol concentration according to Bloor.

All metabolism determinations were performed during hospital admission, the measurements being made in the morning, twelve to fifteen hours after the last meal, using a Krogh closed-circuit type of apparatus. The patients had received the ordinary diet of the ward on the days previous to the determination. For calculation of the metabolism values from the observed oxygen consumption the formulas of Harris and Benedict were used. As a rule, two to six determinations were performed on each patient on separate days, and the lowest of the measurements, if in agreement with the others, accepted as the basal metabolism of the individual.

3. REMARKS CONCERNING THE NUMERICAL TREATMENT OF THE MATERIAL

The data from the case history and the clinical observations for the individual patients were entered in tables which have been subjoined (Tables I—XIII). In these tables the presence of a symptom is denoted by a plus, while the absence of the symptom is marked by a 0. In some instances conclusive information is lacking; if so the place in the table is left blank. The number of unascertained symptoms amounts to 17.3 p.c. for the case history data and to 11.3 p.c. for the physical observations. The percentage occurrence of the symptoms was throughout calculated from the available number of conclusive observations.[1])

For the purpose of numerical and statistic calculations the symptoms have further been entered on punch cards. These punch cards were treated in the usual way in the computations.

As will appear from the following it has occasionally been necessary to omit some of the symptoms in the statistical treatment of the numerical material. Where this has been required, information will be given as to the lines followed in the omission of the symptoms. In some instances the principle has been to avoid including symptoms on which the delimitation of clinical groups of diseases had been based, or which must be regarded as a direct consequence of the primary disease.

It should be noted that in treating so large a numerical material the occurrence of apparent correlations which are a result of accidental coincidences cannot be avoided.

---

[1]) The data given for the frequency of oligomenorrhoea have been computed on the basis of the number of women in the age groups before the menopause.

4. SUBDIVISION OF THE HYPOMETABOLISM MATERIAL

From Table 1 it will be seen how a clinical division of the patients with hypometabolism into 5 main groups and 16 subgroups has been possible. The 5 main groups, comprising in all 11 of the subgroups, were termed: Genuine Myxedema, Reduced Activity, Reduced Intake of Nourishment, Hypogonadism, and Uncertain Cases. It should be noted, however, that a division of the material on other lines is also conceivable, and that some of the patients may with equal propriety be referred to two or more of the groups set up.

TABLE 1

Survey of hypometabolism material.

		Number of Patients
I. Genuine Myxedema	1. Genuine myxedema	18
	2. Congenital myxedema	1
	3. Hypometabolism following treatment of Graves' disease	11
II. Reduced Activity	4. Invalidating polyarthritis	10
	5. Prolonged treatment in bed, or convalescence	11
	6. Organic diseases of the nervous system	18
	7. Chronic intoxication caused by morphine preparations or barbiturates	5
III. Reduced Intake of Nourishment	8. Loss of weight, and subnutrition	22
	9. Nervous anorexia	13
	10. Vomiting due to organic diseases	4
	11. Vegetarian diet through several years	2
IV. Hypogonadism	12. Hypogonadism	64
	13. Psychoses, and severe mental depressions	15
	14. Sclerodermia	1
	15. Amputations of extremities	4
V. Uncertain Cases	16. Uncertain cases of hypometabolism	109
	Total	308

From the table it appears that only 18 of the 308 patients, or barely 6 p.c., were suffering from genuine myxedema with classical changes of the skin of the face (Group 1). In this connection it must be pointed out, however, that in selecting the patients for this group great stress was laid on the certainty of the diagnosis. In one case (Group 2) the myxedema had persisted since the earliest infancy.

It will further be seen from the table that in 11 cases a reduced metabolic rate was demonstrated in patients who had previously suffered from Graves' disease or inflammation of the thyroid gland (Group 3). The majority of these patients had several years before admission to the Holstebro District Hospital undergone subtotal thyroidectomy or X-ray radiation of the thyroid gland as a treatment for Graves' disease; only in 2 of the patients of this group (Nos. 23 and 26) had the hyperthyroidism disappeared during an exclusively medical therapy. Even though it cannot be regarded as proved that the reduction in the metabolic rate demonstrated was in all the patients connected with the thyroid affection from which they had previously suffered, or with its treatment, it was nevertheless considered correct to segregate these patients in a special group.

In 44 cases or in 14 p.c. it must be supposed that the hypometabolism must have been due to a reduction in the activity of the patients. In 10 patients the cause was the presence of a serious polyarthritis with a reduced mobility of the joints (Group 4), in 11 patients confinement to bed for more than one month (Group 5), and in 18 the occurrence of a severe organic nervous disease with associated invalidity or a general debility due to the disease (Group 6). Finally, in 5 patients the decreased activity was caused by the habitual use of morphine or barbiturates in large doses through several years (Group 7).

In the next main group, comprising 41 patients, or 13 p.c. of the patients with hypometabolism, there is a decrease in the intake of food or a marked underweight as the most probable explanation of the reduced metabolic rate. Thus Group 8 includes patients whose body weight, owing to dyspepsia, was more than 25 p.c. below the ideal weight, as well as patients with dyspepsia taking a diet with a much reduced caloric content, and obese patients undergoing dietetic reduction (22 patients in all). Group 9 comprises 13 cases with symptoms of typical nervous anorexia, Group 10 4 patients with frequent vomiting caused by various organic diseases. In this main group we have further considered it justifiable to include 2 cases in which the patients had for years lived on a vegetarian diet with its lower specific dynamic effect (Group 11).

The next group (Group 12) comprises 64 patients suffering from hypogonadism. This group includes patients who had had the ovaries removed by operation or had been subjected to X-ray treatment of the ovaries, as well as young women with scanty menstruation suffering from hot flushes and attacks of sweating and a number of patients with marked climacteric symptoms.

In addition there are two groups of patients in whom affections have been found, in which the pathogenesis of the hypometabolism has not as yet been established, but in which a correlation between the affection and the reduced metabolic rate must, according to the literature, be regarded as likely, thus 15 cases of pronounced psychosis or severe depressions (Group 13) and 1 case of sclerodermia (Group 14).

Again, the table contains 4 cases of amputation of extremities

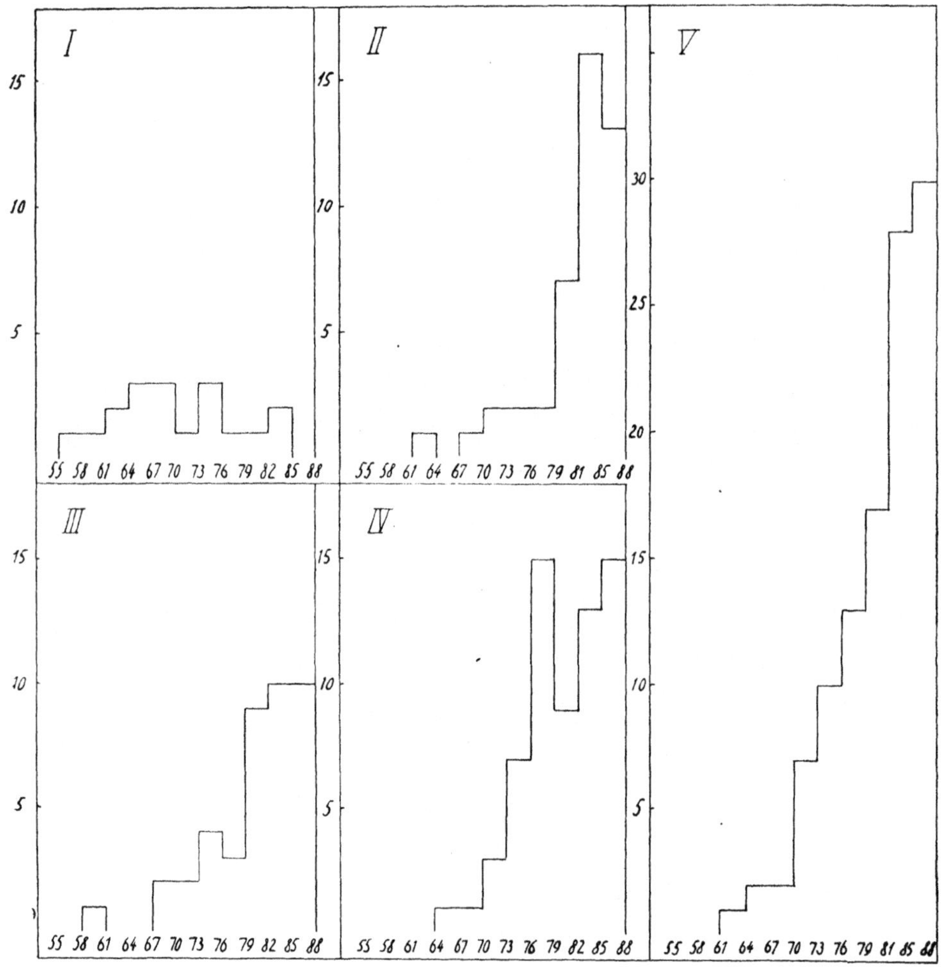

FIG. 3

Graphic representation of observed metabolic values for the individual main groups of hypometabolism. Ordinate: Number of patients. Abscissa: Levels of metabolic rates in per cent of normal.

(Group 15). In these patients the hypometabolism is not real, but is a result of the routine employment of the ordinary calculation tables, no account having been taken in the computation of the metabolic rate of the fact that owing to the amputation the surface of the individuals has been comparatively more reduced than the body weight.

The remaining patients, 109 in all or 36 p.c., have been included in one group which we have called Uncertain Cases; by this we have wished to indicate that the cause of the reduced metabolic rate was not known to us (Group 16).

For illustration of the distribution of the observed metabolic values within the main groups, the values have been represented graphically in Fig. 3.

It will be seen from the plotted curves that the curve representing the cases of genuine myxedema represents a normal distribution curve with a maximum at 71 p.c., while the curves for the other 4 groups seem to correspond to the left section of a distribution curve.

The striking difference between the curve for the cases of genuine myxedema and the curves for the remaining main groups, in the authors' opinion, contributes to emphasise the special position of genuine myxedema among the affections accompanied by hypometabolism. Similar facts have been demonstrated by Means and Lerman (1935) from an American material.

5. SPECIAL FACTS RELATING TO INDIVIDUAL MAIN GROUPS

As stated in the introduction, the data from the case history and the results of the physical examination ascertained for the individual

TABLE 2

The percentage frequency of symptoms in the individual main groups of *men* with hypometabolism.

	Genuine Myxedema	Reduced Activity	Reduced Intake of Nourishment	Hypogonadism	Uncertain Cases	Control Group
	per cent	per cent	per cent	per cent	per cent	per cent
Chilliness	100	50	40	—	70	28
Decreased sweating	50	8	0	—	10	5
Fatigue	100	58	56	—	52	52
Impairment of memory	100	(55)	33	—	24	16
Somnolence	75	22	0	—	21	18
Depression	0	18	38	—	13	11
Dyspepsia	0	17	64	—	21	41
Constipation	100	(25)	(36)	—	9	20
Oliguria	33	0	0	—	0	0
Oligomenorrhoea	—	—	—	—	—	—
Rheumatism	67	(73)	38	—	56	33
Apathy	100	8	9	—	6	5
Depression	0	100	9	—	15	0
Scantiness of hair of scalp	—	—	—	—	—	—
Scantiness of eyebrows	33	0	0	—	10	16
Changes in the skin of the face	(100)	0	0	—	0	0
Hoarseness	100	8	0	—	3	2
Enlargement of the thyroid gland	0	0	0	—	9	4
Scantiness of axillary hair	67	0	17	—	0	5
Scantiness of pubic hair	67	0	0	—	0	5
Thickening of the skin and subcutaneous tissues of the extremities	25	0	0	—	0	0
Perniosis	25	(0)	0	—	3	2
Subcutaneous infiltrations	33	(18)	13	—	17	7
Myalgiae	33	(17)	0	—	39	20
Bradycardia	50	17	27	—	36	21
Hypothermia	0	8	9	—	6	1
Number of patients	4	11	11	—	33	58

patients with hypometabolism will be found in the appended tables (Tables I—XIII), where the division into groups has been retained. With a view to a further statistic treatment of the material we have calculated the percentage frequency of the symptoms within the 5 main groups: Genuine Myxedema, Reduced Activity, Reduced Intake of Nourishment, Hypogonadism, and Uncertain Cases. These calculations were made for men and women separately, as well as for all the patients within the main groups and have been entered in Tables 2, 3, and 4. Further, the tables contain for comparative purposes a numerical statement of the percentage ocurrence of the symptoms in the control material. The figures for the symptoms that have been

TABLE 3

The percentage frequency of symptoms in the individual main groups of *women* with hypometabolism.

	Genuine Myxedema per cent	Reduced Activity per cent	Reduced Intake of Nourishment per cent	Hypogonadism per cent	Uncertain Cases per cent	Control Group per cent
Chilliness	91	64	70	84	74	49
Decreased sweating	72	9	20	21	26	13
Fatigue	100	86	86	92	85	70
Impairment of memory	100	(46)	23	66	27	33
Somnolence	89	26	0	32	35	27
Depression	46	13	22	33	25	22
Dyspepsia	15	7	63	51	25	29
Constipation	93	(68)	(77)	72	43	45
Oliguria	18	4	0	8	5	4
Oligomenorrhoea	67	7	14	(54)	5	17
Rheumatism	91	(73)	63	84	72	60
Apathy	64	13	11	17	13	4
Depression	21	24	12	17	14	5
Scantiness of hair of scalp	83	9	7	14	13	16
Scantiness of eyebrows	75	14	8	43	18	16
Changes in the skin of the face	(100)	0	0	0	4	0
Hoarseness	62	0	4	4	5	4
Enlargement of the thyroid gland	0	0	7	10	13	6
Scantiness of axillary hair	64	10	5	15	10	14
Scantiness of pubic hair	64	14	13	26	13	11
Thickening of the skin and subcutaneous tissues of the extremities	71	3	3	3	4	0
Perniosis	0	(11)	4	31	43	19
Subcutaneous infiltrations	70	(73)	39	69	62	29
Myalgiae	70	(68)	48	66	60	37
Bradycardia	15	6	10	17	17	14
Hypothermia	8	0	0	5	0	1
Number of patients	14	33	30	64	76	132

TABLE 4

The percentage frequency of symptoms in the individual main groups of the *total number of patients* (both men and women) with hypometabolism.

	Genuine Myxedema per cent	Reduced Activity per cent	Reduced Intake of Nourishment per cent	Hypogonadism per cent	Uncertain Cases per cent	Control Group per cent
Chilliness	94	60	64	85	95	43
Decreased sweating	67	9	6	21	20	10
Fatigue	100	78	79	92	75	64
Impairment of memory	100	(47)	25	66	27	28
Somnolence	85	25	0	32	31	24
Depression	39	15	26	33	20	19
Dyspepsia	12	14	63	51	24	32
Constipation	95	(56)	(66)	72	32	38
Oliguria	21	3	0	8	3	3
Oligomenorrhoea	67	7	14	(54)	5	17
Rheumatism	86	(80)	56	86	67	52
Apathy	72	12	10	17	11	4
Depression	18	27	11	17	15	4
Scantiness of hair of scalp	83	9	7	14	13	16
Scantiness of eyebrows	67	9	6	43	16	16
Changes in the skin of the face	(100)	0	0	0	3	0
Hoarseness	50	3	4	4	4	3
Enlargement of the thyroid gland	0	0	5	10	12	5
Scantiness of axillary hair	64	7	7	15	6	11
Scantiness of pubic hair	64	10	10	26	8	10
Thickening of the skin and subcutaneous tissues of the extremities	61	2	3	3	3	0
Perniosis	7	(8)	3	31	29	14
Subcutaneous infiltrations	62	(59)	33	69	48	23
Myalgiae	62	(54)	38	66	54	32
Bradycardia	24	9	15	17	23	16
Hypothermia	6	2	2	5	2	1
Number of patients	18	44	41	64	109	190
Average metabolism (p.c. of normal)	71	83	83	81	80	
Average increment value	829	477	234	365	365	
Average diuresis (ml)	478	486	703	589	595	616
Average cholesterol content of serum in mg per 100 ml	542	253	190	255	190	
Average age at admission to the hospital (years)	52	44	33	37	34	41
Average deviation from the ideal weight (per cent)	+33	+17	—1	+18	+18	+14

determining for the delimitation of a group, or must be supposed to be a direct consequence of the primary affection, are given in paranthesis (thus constipation in long confinement to bed and in insufficient intake of nourishment, and absence of perniosis following prolonged treatment in bed).

Genuine Myxedema.

From Tables 2, 3, and 4 it will appear that a series of symptoms occur with predominant frequency in the group Genuine Myxedema, thus: decreased sweating, fatigue, impairment of memory, sleepiness, constipation, a subjective impression of oliguria, apathy, hoarseness, and scantiness of eyebrows, axillary and pubic hair. We shall later (see p. 32) try to elucidate in how far the symptoms quoted are associated with the hypometabolism or with the myxedematous condition as such. Further we note that the average metabolic rate for this group is essentially lower (71 p.c.) than for the groups Reduced Activity, Reduced Intake of Nourishment, Hypogonadism, and Uncertain Cases (see Table 4 and Fig. 3), while the average serum cholesterol value is more than double the normal value. In the measurement of the diuresis, on the other hand, the presence of oliguria in genuine myxedema could not be numerically established in relation to the other groups. This observation gives rise to some doubt as to the correctness of the information given by the patients concerning the occurrence of oliguria in the group Genuine Myxedema, though the possibility cannot be dismissed that the spontaneous intake of fluid in the home may have been less than the routine intake of fluid at the hospital. In estimating these conditions it must be taken into account whether the patients with genuine myxedema, owing to their state of apathy, void less often in the course of the 24 hours than other patients. If this be the case, the patients may easily confuse the frequency of urination with the amount of the diuresis, as it will presumably be difficult for some patients to distinguish between these concepts.

Hypogonadism.

As mentioned above, the material of patients with hypometabolism contains a very considerable number of persons suffering from hypogonadism, no less than 21 p.c. coming within this group, a fact which does not appear to have been previously noted in the literature,[1]) and which it therefore seems of special interest to the authors to point out. On the basis hereof it must be established that patients with hypogonadism constitute a very essential part of the cases of hypometabolism found in medical departments.

On the other hand, in order to elucidate how great a part hypo-

---

[1]) The authors desire to express their thanks to Professor Eggert Møller who, during the treatment of the material, pointed out the significance of this group.

metabolism plays in the clinical aspect of hypogonadism, the patients with hypogonadism in the control material were enumerated, similar criteria being used in the selection of the patients as in the examination of the hypometabolic material. In this treatment of the control material, 35 patients with hypogonadism were selected among 190 patients, corresponding to 18 p.c. of the control group. 30 out of the 64 patients with hypogonadism in the hypometabolic material date from the same period (February 1, 1941—January 31, 1942). It may then be estimated that about half of the patients with hypogonadism in a medical department will have a reduced metabolic rate, while about half have a normal metabolic rate. In good agreement herewith the average metabolic rate for all the patients with hypogonadism from the period February 1, 1941 to January 31, 1942 was calculated at 89 p.c. (see also Fig. 3).

A perusal of Table 3 will show that a number of symptoms within the group Hypogonadism occur with essentially greater frequency than in the female patients of the control group, thus: chilliness, fatigue, impairment of memory, dyspepsia, constipation, scantiness of eyebrows, perniosis, subcutaneous infiltrations, and myalgiae. This shows that, apart from the characteristic skin changes of the face, there is a certain similarity to the symptoms for the group genuine myxedema, since in this disease too, as stated in the table and previously mentioned, the symptoms fatigue, impairment of memory, constipation, and scantiness of eyebrows occur with particular frequency. The dyspepsia which has been observed in half of the patients with hypogonadism is presumably in many cases secondary to the constipation.

The observed similarity between the symptoms in genuine myxedema and in hypogonadism would seem to support the supposition that the symptoms in hypogonadism might at any rate in part be due to a secondary hypothyroidism. If this were the case, a considerable clinical improvement might be expected from thyroid medication, but as will presently be shown in the section on the results of thyroid administration, the effect of thyroid in hypogonadism is not any greater than in the other main groups of non-myxedematous reduction of the metabolic rate.

It has been mentioned above that in about half of the patients with hypogonadism admitted to a medical department a reduction of the basal metabolism may be anticipated. In order to decide whether there is any difference, in a clinical investigation on the lines laid down in this work, between the symptoms of patients suffering from hypogonadism with a normal metabolism and with a reduced metabolic rate, a comparison has been made in Table 5 between the percentage frequencies of the symptoms within these two groups. In this table the values for the 64 patients with hypogonadism from the hypometabolism material (Table 3, Column 4) are compared with the

TABLE 5

The percentage frequency of symptoms in women suffering from hypogonadism associated with hypometabolism, and with a normal metabolic rate.

Metabolic rate in per cent	≦ 88	> 88
Chilliness	84	47
Decreased sweating	21	6
Fatigue	92	71
Impairment of memory	66	34
Somnolence	32	29
Depression	33	26
Dyspepsia	51	40
Constipation	72	51
Oliguria	5	3
Oligomenorrhoea	54	89
Rheumatism	84	55
Apathy	17	0
Depression	17	0
Scantiness of hair of scalp	14	9
Scantiness of eyebrows	43	17
Changes in the skin of the face	0	0
Hoarseness	4	3
Enlargement of the thyroid gland	10	3
Scantiness of axillary hair	15	21
Scantiness of pubic hair	26	15
Thickening of the skin and subcutaneous tissues of the extremities	3	0
Perniosis	31	17
Subcutaneous infiltrations	69	31
Myalgiae	66	37
Bradycardia	17	14
Hypothermia	4	3
Number of patients	64	35

calculated percentage values for the 35 patients with hypogonadism from the control group.

Such a comparison shows that no less than 12 of the symptoms, namely chilliness, decreased sweating, fatigue, impaired memory, constipation, apathy, depression, scantiness of eyebrows, scantiness of pubic hair, perniosis, subcutaneous infiltrations, and myalgiae occur with predominant frequency in the patients with hypogonadism in whom a metabolic rate of 88 p.c. or less has been demonstrated. In estimating this finding it must, however, be taken into account that the majority of these symptoms (chilliness, fatigue, constipation, apathy, depression, scantiness of eyebrows, perniosis, subcutaneous infiltrations, and myalgiae), as will appear from the results presented in a later section, seem to be associated with the reduced basal metabolism as such.

Uncertain Cases.

In a large group of patients comprising 109 cases, or more than one third of all the patients with hypometabolism who were examined, we were, as already mentioned, unable to ascertain the cause of the reduced metabolic rate, and this is the reason why this group has been called Uncertain Cases, despite the fact that for most of the patients a reliable clinical diagnosis was available. For the sake of clarity the diagnoses for these patients have been given in Table 6.

TABLE 6

Survey of clinical diagnoses for the main group Uncertain Cases, comprising 109 patients.

Arterial hypertension	1
Arthritis	2
Asthenia	2
Brachial neuralgia	1
Cardiac neurosis	5
Cerebral arteriosclerosis	1
Cholelithiasis	4
Chronic bursitis	1
Chronic colitis	1
Chronic constipation	9
Coronary sclerosis	3
Eczema	3
Epilepsy	1
Hysteria	1
Myalgia	9
Neurasthenia	15
Normal	21
Obesity	19
Oligophrenia	2
Prolapse of intervertebral disc	2
Syphilis	2
Valvular aortic disease	1

The very interesting fact emerging from the table is that in 21 of the 109 patients contained in this group there were no signs of disease at all, so these individuals must be regarded as healthy. This observation seems to the authors to afford essential evidence which warrants the positing of the concept "physiological hypometabolism". In other words, in a number of individuals it will be possible to ascertain a reduced basal metabolism as a non-pathological finding, a fact which, besides being of theoretical interest, has a considerable practical significance, both in a diagnostic and a therapeutic respect. Thus the finding of a reduced basal metabolism may be anticipated in a number of cases in connection with the clinical examination of hospitalised patients; from this the mistake may arise to regard the hypometabolism as a part of the patient's primary disease.

The observed metabolic values for the above-mentioned 21 patients ranged from 70 to 86 p.c.; the average metabolic value was 81 p.c.. On the basis hereof it can be established that in some healthy individuals metabolic rates may be observed that are considerably lower than the normal values usually given.

For the further study of the question as to the occurrence of a physiological hypometabolism, Professor Eggert Møller, Copenhagen, has suggested that we should enter all the metabolic rates in the group Uncertain Cases from the period February 1, 1941 to January 31, 1942 (a total of 58 patients) in a graph and compare this graph to a curve of the metabolic values for the control cases from the same one-year period (a total of 190 patients). If these two curves together form the left and the right section respectively of a distribution curve

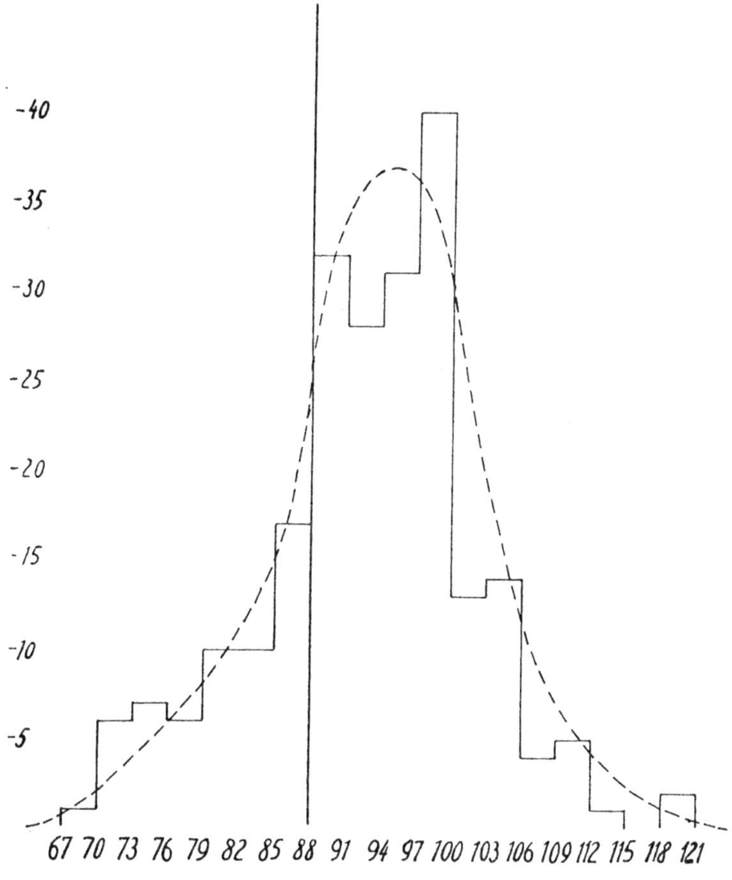

FIG. 4

Graphic representation of metabolic values for the main group Uncertain Cases from the period February 1, 1941 to January 31, 1942 (left section of figure) and the Patients of the Control Group from the same one-year period (right section of figure). Ordinate: Number of patients. Abscissa: Levels of metabolic rates in per cent of normal.

this will render it probable that for some non-normal individuals too in the group Uncertain Cases we are merely concerned with a normal variation. As will appear from Fig. 4, the curves, when joined together, actually do form a distribution curve with the maximum at 94 p.c.[1]). Thus this finding supports the assumption that the observed hypometabolism in no small number of medical patients is no pathological symptom. In this connection it should be mentioned that in 1935 Means and Lerman published a curve of the distribution of metabolic rates for patients in whom the clinical examination revealed no signs of thyroid affections. This curve which, however, also includes groups not entering into the material for the curve in Fig. 4, likewise shows a maximum at a metabolic rate of 94 p.c..

[1]) A curve for the metabolic values for the Uncertain Cases from *the whole three-year period* will be seen in Fig. 3.

6. RELATION OF THE SYMPTOMS TO THE SEX AND AGE OF THE PATIENTS

The total hypometabolism material (with the exception of the cases in Group 15, the patients who had had extremities amputated) has been statistically treated with a view to ascertaining the correlation of the symptoms to the *sex* of the patients. This treatment, as will appear too from a comparison between Tables 2 and 3, shows that only one of the symptoms, bradycardia, occurs more frequently in men than in women, while a large number of symptoms: chilliness, fatigue, constipation, scantiness of eyebrows and pubic hair, perniosis, subcutaneous infiltrations, and myalgiae occur chiefly in women.

Further, the correlation between the frequency of the symptoms and the *age* of the patients has been subjected to statistic investigation for all the symptoms in the female patients[1]). This analysis showed (see Table 7) that impaired memory, scantiness of the hair of the scalp, eyebrows, axillary and pubic hair, as well as subcutaneous infiltrations and myalgiae occur more frequently in the higher age classes, while perniosis appears with decreasing frequency in the elderly patients. As far as the other symptoms are concerned it was not possible to demonstrate any correlation with the age of the patients.

---

[1]) In these calculations the authors did not extend the numerical investigations to the total hypometabolism material, but confined themselves to the female patients because of the correlation noted in the preceding paragraph between a series of symptoms and the sex of the patients.

TABLE 7

Relation of the symptoms to the age of the patients (Observations on female patients only).

Age in years	16—25	26—35	36—45	46—55	56—65	66—75
	per cent	per cent	per cent	per cent	per cent	per cent
Chilliness	68	75	78	80	82	50
Decreased sweating	17	24	45	8	33	0
Fatigue	82	88	88	95	96	88
Impairment of memory	10	37	69	78	77	50
Somnolence	31	36	48	39	25	12
Depression	25	26	43	39	22	0
Dyspepsia	28	38	47	35	19	22
Constipation	42	68	66	69	85	56
Oliguria	2	7	6	13	10	0
Oligomenorrhoea	23	20	27	—	—	—
Rheumatism	58	67	91	95	100	77
Apathy	27	9	19	23	24	11
Depression	18	12	26	16	9	22
Scantiness of hair of scalp	5	15	14	26	44	17
Scantiness of eyebrows	10	10	41	57	59	33
Changes in the skin of the face	3	2	8	14	27	0
Hoarseness	4	4	9	13	14	0
Enlargement of the thyroid gland	17	18	80	7	4	0
Scantiness of axillary hair	6	0	18	26	41	33
Scantiness of pubic hair	12	12	22	33	47	16
Thickening of the skin and subcutaneous tissues of the extremities	3	4	3	16	27	0
Perniosis	45	25	24	9	5	0
Subcutaneous infiltrations	39	42	80	87	96	89
Myalgiae	32	49	84	82	88	89
Bradycardia	18	15	5	18	4	22
Hypothermia	5	2	3	0	0	0
Number of patients	65	60	38	45	28	7

7. RELATION OF THE SYMPTOMS TO THE REDUCED BASAL METABOLISM AND THE DEGREE OF REDUCTION

The numerical material given in Table 3 has been treated with a view to ascertaining whether it is possible to decide if any of the symptoms are associated with the hypometabolism as such. The treat-

TABLE 8
Comparison of the percentage frequency of the symptoms in women with non-myxedematous hypometabolism, and in the control group.

	Non-myxedematous Hypometabolism per cent	Control Group per cent
Chilliness	75	49
Decreased sweating	21	13
Fatigue	87	70
Impairment of memory	44	33
Somnolence	29	27
Depression	25	22
Dyspepsia	36	29
Constipation	61	45
Oliguria	5	4
Oligomenorrhoea	21	17
Rheumatism	77	60
Apathy	14	4
Depression	22	5
Scantiness of hair of scalp	12	16
Scantiness of eyebrows	24	16
Changes in the skin of the face	2	0
Hoarseness	3	4
Enlargement of the thyroid gland	9	6
Scantiness of axillary hair	10	14
Scantiness of pubic hair	17	11
Thickening of the skin and subcutaneous tissues of the extremities	4	0
Perniosis	28	19
Subcutaneous infiltrations	63	29
Myalgiae	61	37
Bradycardia	14	14
Hypothermia	2	1
Number of patients	243	132

ment comprises the female patients[1]) within the main groups Reduced Activity, Reduced Intake of Nourishment, Hypogonadism, Uncertain Cases, and the Control Group, whereas the patients with Genuine Myxedema have not been included on account of the special position of this group. For the sake of clarity the authors have assembled in a special table (Table 8) the above-mentioned 4 main groups of patients with hypometabolism from Table 3 and entered the control group from Table 3 for comparison. From this comparison it appears that a large number of symptoms (12): chilliness, decreased sweating, fatigue, im-

TABLE 9

Relation of the percentage frequency of the symptoms to the level of metabolic rate. (Observations on female patients only).

Metabolic rate in per cent	≦ 78	79-83	84-88	89-93	94-103	≧ 104
Chilliness	76	73	71	37	53	58
Decreased sweating	25	23	14	13	13	11
Fatigue	89	91	83	74	70	63
Impairment of memory	60	37	30	28	28	41
Somnolence	39	40	29	16	30	33
Depression	33	26	27	23	19	30
Dyspepsia	39	35	31	38	26	22
Constipation	75	55	55	40	43	44
Oliguria	9	5	3	0	7	4
Oligomenorrhoea	32	14	23	17	17	0
Rheumatism	74	73	77	65	58	55
Apathy	25	12	15	3	6	0
Depression	18	9	28	5	7	0
Scantiness of hair of scalp	16	3	17	13	16	33
Scantiness of eyebrows	31	26	18	18	16	11
Changes in the skin of the face	0	2	2	0	0	0
Hoarseness	2	2	5	0	6	4
Enlargement of the thyroid gland	7	6	13	5	6	7
Scantiness of axillary hair	18	8	7	13	12	19
Scantiness of pubic hair	15	18	18	13	9	21
Thickening of the skin and subcutaneous tissues of the extremities	0	3	6	0	0	0
Perniosis	15	36	23	15	21	18
Subcutaneous infiltrations	52	64	66	31	29	26
Myalgiae	56	63	62	38	38	33
Bradycardia	31	10	7	21	13	11
Hypothermia	4	0	2	3	0	0
Number of patients	72	75	96	36	62	34

[1]) For the reasons stated in the footnote on page 27, these calculations were limited to the female patients.

pairment of memory, constipation, rheumatism, objective apathy and depression, scantiness of eyebrows, perniosis, subcutaneous infiltrations, and myalgiae occur with statistically greater frequency within the female hypometabolism groups in question than in the female patients with a normal metabolism.

The female hypometabolism material examined has further been classed according to the metabolic rates measured, and the frequency of the symptoms noted for the metabolic rates ≦ 78 p.c., 79—83 p.c., 84—88 p.c., 89—93 p.c., 94—103 p.c., ≧ 104 p.c. (Table 9).

The table shows that the above-mentioned 12 symptoms which oc-

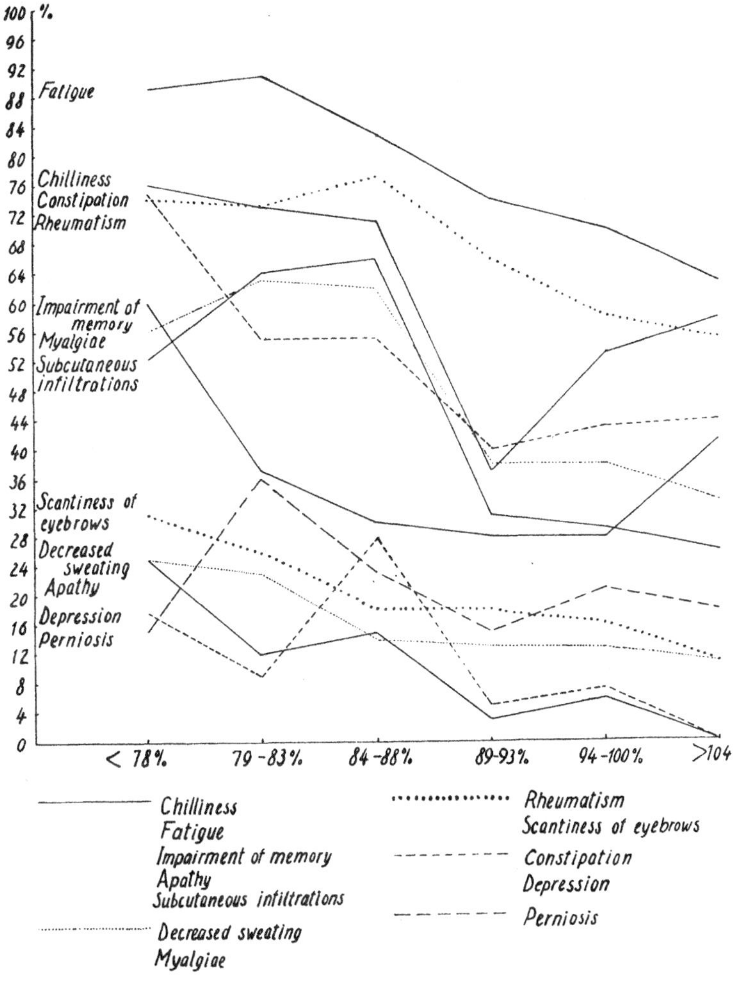

FIG. 5

Graphic representation of the percentage frequency of a series of symptoms at various metabolic levels. Ordinate: Percentage frequency of the symptoms. Abscissa: Metabolic rates in per cent of normal.

curred with greater frequency within the hypometabolism groups than within the control group, as a rule occur with greater frequency at the lowest metabolic rates, so that on the whole a handsome correlation may be observed between the percentage occurrence of the symptoms in question and the degree of reduction of the basal metabolism. A graphic representation of this finding is shown in Fig. 5.

A special contribution to the elucidation of the difference in the

TABLE 10
Comparison of symptoms in genuine myxedema and in non-myxedematous hypometabolism.

	Genuine Myxedema	Hypometabolism
Chilliness	+	+
Decreased sweating	+	+
Fatigue	+	+
Impairment of memory	+	+
Somnolence	+	
Constipation	+	+
Oliguria	+	
Rheumatism	+	+
Apathy	+	+
Depression	+	+
Scantiness of hair of scalp	+	
Scantiness of eyebrows	+	+
Changes in the skin of the face	+	
Hoarseness	+	
Scantiness of axillary hair	+	
Scantiness of pubic hair	+	
Thickening of the skin and subcutaneous tissues of the extremities	+	
Perniosis		+
Subcutaneous infiltrations	+	+
Myalgiae	+	+

symptoms for genuine myxedema and for non-myxedematous hypometabolism was finally obtained by comparing the symptoms found for genuine myxedema (see the first column of Table 3 and p. 21) and the 12 symptoms mentioned on p. 30 which seem to be associated with the reduction of the basal metabolism. From this comparison (see Table 10) it appears that only the symptoms: somnolence, skin changes of the face and the extremities, scantiness of the hair of the scalp, and of the axillary and pubic hair, as well as hoarseness can with any great probability be designated as characteristic of genuine myxedema, since for reasons previously stated (see p. 21) it was thought correct to disregard the information given about the subjective impression of oliguria.

8. INVESTIGATIONS ON THE OCCURRENCE AND COMBINATION OF A NUMBER OF SYMPTOMS IN NON-MYXEDEMATOUS PATIENTS WITH REDUCED BASAL METABOLISM AND IN THE CONTROL GROUP

A CONTRIBUTION TO THE ELUCIDATION OF THE SYMPTOMATOLOGY FOR NON-MYXEDEMATOUS HYPOMETABOLISM

When we mentioned the correlation of the symptoms with the reduced metabolism we made numerical determination of the percentage frequency of the symptoms in the control material and in the patients with non-myxedematous hypometabolism (see p. 29, Table 8)[1]. A perusal of the table will show that 10 of the symptoms entered there, namely chilliness, decreased sweating, impairment of memory, constipation, objective apathy, objective depression, scantiness of eyebrows, perniosis, subcutaneous infiltrations, and myalgiae occur more than 33 p.c. oftener in patients with a reduced basal metabolism than in the control group.

In order to investigate more closely the occurrence of these 10 symptoms the authors have for each of the female patients within the hypometabolism group (with the exception of the groups genuine myxedema and amputations of extremities) and within the control group noted down how many and which of the 10 symptoms were found. From the tabulated symptoms the number of symptoms present for each patient has been summed up and the frequency of the combination of 2,3, or 4 symptoms in all the combinations occurring has been calculated.

The result of the summation is entered in Table 11 which shows that in the patients with a reduced basal metabolism there as a rule occurs a larger number of the symptoms quoted than in the patients in the control group.

---

[1]) For the reasons stated in the footnote on p. 27, these calculations were limited to the female patients.

TABLE 11

Occurrence of 10 selected symptoms in women with non-myxedematous hypometabolism and in the control group.

	Non-myxedematous hypometabolism		Control Group	
	Number of patients	per cent	Number of patients	per cent
0 symptom	12	5	17	13
1 symptom	22	9	25	19
2 symptoms	36	15	32	23
3 symptoms	46	19	19	14
4 symptoms	44	18	20	15
5 symptoms	41	17	13	10
6 symptoms	27	11	5	4
7 symptoms	12	5	1	1
8 symptoms	2	1	0	0
9 symptoms	1	0	0	0
10 symptoms	0	0	0	0

On reviewing the above-mentioned 10 symptoms with regard to their combination according to the above-stated principles, the authors have for each of the possible symptom combinations calculated the percentage frequency with which the combination occurs within the hypometabolism group and within the control group. After this the percentages emerging were compared and a certain selection was made of the symptom combinations that occurred with essentially greater frequency in the hypometabolism group than in the control group.

The result of this thoroughgoing numerical treatment is given in Table 12, which shows the frequency of most of the symptom combinations thus selected within the hypometabolism group and within the control group. In this connection it should be noted that the symptoms scantiness of eyebrows and perniosis are not included in the table owing to the fact that combinations into which these symptoms enter do not occur with sufficient predominance within the hypometabolism group.

In the authors' opinion the combinations of symptoms stated here may make an important contribution to the elucidation of the symptomatology of hypometabolism. But, as previously pointed out, it must be kept in mind in estimating the results that in treating such a considerable numerical material it will not be possible to avoid accidental coupling of observations. As a whole, however, the published material must be said to be well suited for elucidating the clinical aspects of hypometabolism.

The authors are anxious to emphasise that even though the figures published in Table 12 serve to throw light on the symptomatology of hypometabolism and also to give a certain indication with regard to the probability of the occurrence of a reduced basal metabolism, the figures given by no means warrant a statement as to the numerical probability of the presence of a reduced metabolic rate on the basis

TABLE 12

Frequency of combinations of 8 selected symptoms in women with non-myxedematous hypometabolism and in the control group.

Chilliness	Decreased sweating	Impairment of memory	Constipation	Apathy	Depression	Subcutaneous infiltrations	Myalgiae	Percentage frequency	
								Hypo-metabolism	Normal metabolic rate
■	■		■				■	5	2
■		■	■			■		14	5
■		■	■				■	14	6
■		■				■		18	6
■		■				■	■	18	4
■		■					■	17	8
■			■					43	20
■			■			■		28	9
■			■			■	■	22	6
■			■				■	29	10
■				■				9	2
■					■			8	2
■						■		40	17
■						■	■	31	14
	■	■				■		6	2
		■	■			■		19	7
		■	■				■	20	9
		■			■			7	2
		■				■		25	10
		■				■	■	22	7
			■		■			8	0
			■			■		37	15
			■			■	■	31	9
			■				■	37	16
				■		■		10	2
				■			■	8	1
					■	■		8	2
					■	■	■	7	0
					■		■	9	1
						■	■	47	20

of the symptoms observed in the individual patient. This would require a knowledge of the percentage frequency of hypometabolism in the population in question. For even if a combination occurs in a high percentage of persons with a reduced basal metabolism and only rarely in individuals with a normal metabolism, the large number of persons with a normal metabolism will render it possible for the absolute number of normal individuals with the symptom combination in question within a population group to be just as large or larger than the number of persons with hypometabolism who present the same combination. It is undoubtedly for this reason that despite the demonstrated considerable difference in the percentage occurrence of the symptom combinations given in Table 12, it has not yet been possible to point out clinical symptoms on an empirical basis which will justify the diagnosis non-myxedematous hypometabolism.

9. INVESTIGATIONS ON THE EFFECT OF THYROID ADMINISTRATION TO PATIENTS WITH HYPOMETABOLISM

In order to ascertain the effect of thyroid administration a treatment with standardised thyroid tablets made of dried powdered thyroid gland obtained from cattle was instituted in those cases in which a therapeutic effect could be expected or could not be regarded as excluded. The tablets used in the treatment were chiefly such as contained an amount of hormone corresponding to 0.4 mg thyroxine, the daily dose being usually 1 tablet. In rare cases a daily dose corresponding to 0.1 or 0.2 mg thyroxine was administered.

Treatment with thyroid has been tried in 135 of the 308 patients with hypometabolism. In 8 of these cases the period of observation was, however, too short to enable us to estimate the effect of the thyroid medication. The observed result of the treatment for the remaining 127 patients is entered at the bottom of the appended tables, the results of the treatment being stated both for the objective and the subjective symptoms. In estimating the objective symptoms special significance has been attached to the evacuation frequency of the bowels, the condition of the skin and hair, and the general appearance, and for the subjective symptoms, changes in fatigue, chilliness, indisposition, and sleepiness. In those cases in which, despite cautious thyroid dosing, an aggravation of the clinical condition occurred, this consisted in the majority of the cases in subjective cardiac symptoms (palpitations, tachycardia, anginoid attacks), as well as attacks of sweating, tremor, and nervousness. In patients presenting symptoms of gastric and duodenal ulcers or with a history of gastric complaints with hyperacidity, we have, however, not rarely observed either an exacerbation of an already existing dyspepsia or the appearance of epigastric pains during the treatment with thyroid. The total results of the treatment of patients from the main groups are given in Table 13. From this it will appear that while objective as well as subjective improvement was obtained after administration in practically all the cases of genuine myxedema, only about 20 p.c. of the rest of the patients with hypometabolism showed objective improvement, and about 35 p.c. subjective improvement. It is further

TABLE 13

Effect of thyroid administration to patients with hypometabolism.

Main Group	Number of treated patients	Effect of Treatment: Objective Symptoms: Improved per cent	Objective Symptoms: Unchanged per cent	Objective Symptoms: Aggravated per cent	Subjective Symptoms: Improved per cent	Subjective Symptoms: Unchanged per cent	Subjective Symptoms: Aggravated per cent
Genuine Myxedema	18	94	6	0	100	0	0
Reduced Activity	10	30	70	0	30	70	0
Reduced Intake of Nourishment	7	0	100	0	29	42	29
Hypogonadism	42	21	79	0	29	52	19
Uncertain Cases	52	21	79	0	42	50	8

seen from Table 13 that the patients within the separate groups of non-myxedematous reduction of the metabolic rate exhibit fairly uniform conditions in this respect. It must be pointed out that in estimating the results of the treatment the observation of an improvement following the administration of thyroid does not necessarily warrant the conclusion that the patient is suffering from myxedema, since the rise in the metabolic rate accompanying the administration of thyroid may in itself cause an improvement in the general condition of the patients (e.g. by the cessation of chilliness). The laxative effect that can frequently be observed in normal individuals upon the administration of thyroid may undoubtedly also occur in some cases of hypometabolism, without the constipation being for that reason due to a thyroid deficiency. From Table 13 it will appear that an aggravation of the clinical condition following thyroid administration was observed in 0 cases, or 0 p.c., for the objective symptoms, and in 14 cases, or 10 p.c., for the subjective symptoms.

A review of the data showing the frequency with which the clinical symptoms found upon admission occur in patients with non-myxedematous hypometabolism whose condition improved objectively during thyroid administration, compared with patients whose condition remained unchanged or was aggravated, shows no conclusive difference (see Table 14). The patients' subjective impression of the effect of the treatment likewise seems unrelated to the symptoms present prior to the thyroid medication. This observation is of practical interest, seeing that it seems to be impossible, according to the results here communicated, to form any conclusive idea from the clinical symptoms presented by patients with non-myxedematous hypometabolism as to whether a proposed thyroid medication may be expected to cause an improvement or not.

It further appears from the table that the height of the metabolic rate at the institution of the treatment shows no correlation to the result of the treatment.

TABLE 14

The percentage frequency of symptoms in untreated patients with non-myxedematous hypometabolism, improved and unimproved following thyroid administration.

	Objective Symptoms		Subjective Symptoms	
	Improved	Unchanged	Improved	Unchanged or Aggravated
Chilliness	80	80	80	79
Decreased sweating	33	25	45	17
Fatigue	100	94	90	99
Impairment of memory	37	63	42	66
Somnolence	54	39	53	31
Depression	22	33	40	28
Dyspepsia	25	35	26	40
Constipation	86	69	60	78
Oliguria	5	11	11	6
Oligomenorrhoea	25	24	17	28
Rheumatism	89	85	86	87
Apathy	14	22	17	22
Depression	0	21	19	15
Scantiness of hair of scalp	11	17	8	19
Scantiness of eyebrows	11	38	22	35
Changes in the skin of the face	0	2	0	3
Hoarseness	5	3	8	2
Enlargement of the thyroid gland	9	17	13	16
Scantiness of axillary hair	0	12	8	10
Scantiness of pubic hair	0	20	8	18
Thickening of the skin and subcutaneous tissues of the extremities	0	6	3	5
Perniosis	44	38	48	33
Subcutaneous infiltrations	64	75	77	76
Myalgiae	57	34	46	66
Bradycardia	18	19	16	20
Hypothermia	0	1	0	1
Number of patients	22	90	30	82
Average metabolism (per cent)	80	80	80	79

For the purpose of further investigation of the effect of the thyroid administration the capability of the thyroid administration to raise the metabolic rate was investigated. In order to arrive at a numerical expression of this relation the "increment value" for the individual thyroid-treated patients was calculated according to the principles indicated by Møller in 1926. In this calculation the following equation was used:

$$\text{Increment value} = \frac{\text{Increase in metabolic rate in per cent}}{\text{Thyroxine dose per kg body weight in tenths of a milligram}}$$

The calculated mean increment values for the separate main groups are given at the bottom of Table 4. The table shows the interesting fact that the mean increment value for the patients in the group Genuine Myxedema is more than double the amount of the mean increment value for the rest of the cases, a finding which (similarly to the increased mean serum cholesterol value and the graphs indicating the distribution of the metabolic values) stresses the special position of genuine myxedema.

The results we have communicated emphasise the necessity of trying to classify the cause of the hypometabolism before a thyroid treatment is considered. The requirements laid down for the delimitation of the group genuine myxedema were, as already mentioned, very strict, and it cannot be excluded that among the remaining patients with hypometabolism there may have been cases of mild myxedema.

In some instances, therefore, where classical skin changes do not occur it may presumably be indicated to try the effect of a thyroid therapy. In such cases the calculated increment value may be of importance for the decision of the justification of a continued thyroid administration. Often observation under hospital conditions will be necessary.

From the results communicated in this exposition it will appear that for an adequate treatment of the patients' complaints other therapeutic measures will frequently be required than thyroid treatment, e.g. correction of the state of nourishment, administration of estrogen compounds etc..

In conclusion we should like once more to emphasise that the reduction of the metabolic rate in a great number of patients in a medical department must be regarded as a non-pathological finding or as a symptom which does not reveal hypothyroidism, so that in these cases a treatment with thyroid cannot be regarded as indicated.

REFERENCES

Boothby, W. M., and Sandiford, I., Summary of the basal metabolism data on 8.614 subjects with especial reference to the normal standards for the estimation of the basal metabolic rate. J. Biol. Chem., *54*, 783, 1922.

Carpenter, T., Tables, factors and formulas for computing respiratory exchange and biological transformations of energy. Carnegie Institution of Washington. Publication No. 303. 1921.

Cecil, R. L., Barr, D. P., and Du Bois, E. F., Clinical calorimetry XXXI. Observations on the metabolism of arthritis. Arch. Int. Med., *29*, 583, 1922.

Du Bois, E. F., Basal metabolism in health and disease. Lea and Febiger. Philadelphia. 1927.

Haines, S. F., and Mussey, R. D., Certain menstrual disturbances associated with low basal metabolic rates without myxedema. J. A. M. A., *105*, 557, 1935.

Harris, J. A., and Benedict, F. G., A biometric study of basal metabolism in man. Carnegie Institution of Washington. Publication No. 279. 1919.

Hoskins, R. G., Oxygen consumption (»Basal metabolic rate«) in schizophrenia. II. Distributions in two hundred and fourteen cases. Arch. Neurol. and Psychiat., *28*, 1346, 1932.

Krogh, A., Ein Respirationsapparat zur klinischen Bestimmung des Energieumsatzes des Menschen. Wien. klin. Wchnschr., *35*, 290, 1922.

Longcope, .W. T., Hypoglycemia in scleroderma. The metabolism in eight cases with reference to the function of the glands of internal secretion. J. A. M. A., *90*, 1, 1928.

Lusk, G., The physiological effect of undernutrition. Physiol. Rev., *1*, 523, 1921.

Means, J. H., The thyroid and its diseases. J. B. Lippincott Co. Philadelphia. 1937.

Means, J. H., and Lerman, J., The symptomatology of myxedema. Its relation to metabolic levels, time intervals and rations of thyroid. Arch. Int. Med., *55*, 1, 1935.

Møller, E., Clinical investigations into the basal metabolism in diseases of the thyroid gland. Acta med. Scandinav., Supplement. 21, 1927.

— Rapports quantitatifs du métabolisme dans la dénutrition. Ann. de méd., *16*, 451, 1924.

Pemberton, R., and Tompkins, E. H., Studies on arthritis in the army based on four hundred cases. II. Observations on the basal metabolism. Arch. Int. med., *25*, 241, 1920.

Peters, J. P., and Van Slyke, D. D., Quantitative Clinical Chemistry. The William & Wilkins Co., Baltimore. 1931.

Seward, B. P., A clinical study of the mild grades of hypothyroidism. Ann. Int. Med., *9*, 178, 1935.

APPENDED TABLES
CLINICAL NOTES AND CASE HISTORY NUMBERS FOR PATIENTS WITH HYPOMETABOLISM

Clinical Data for the Individual Patients with Hypometabolism

TABLE I

	1. Genuine myxedema																				2. Congenital myxedema			3. Hypometabolism following treatment of Graves' disease			
	1	2	3	4	5	6	7	8	9	10	11	12	13	14	15	16	17	18			19			20	21	22	
	F	F	F	F	F	M	F	F	M	M	F	F	F	F	F	F	F	F			F			F	F	F	
	62	59	36	55	39	62	51	46	23	61	49	64	54	65	48	56	59	51			31			34	33	48	
	C	C	T	C	C	C	T	C	C	C	C	C	C	T	C	C	T	C			C			T	C	C	
1	+	+	+	+		+	+	+	+	+	+	+	o	+	+	+	+	+						+	+	o	1
2	o	+	+		+				+	o				+	o	+									o	o	2
3	+	+	+	+	+	+	+	+	+	+	+	+	+	+	+	+	+	+			+				+	+	3
4	+	+	+	+	+	+	+		+	+	+		+	+		+	+	+			+				+	+	4
5	+	+	+	+	+	o	+		+	+				+	+	o		+							+	o	5
6	o	+	+	o		o	+				+		o	o	+	o	o	o			+				o	o	6
7	+	o	o		o	o	+	o	o	o	o	o	o	o	o	o	o	o						o	o	o	7
8	+	+	+	+	+	+	+	+	+	+	+	+	+	+	o	+	+	+			+			+	+	o	8
9	o	+	o		o	o		o	+	o	+		o	o	o	o	o				o				o	o	9
10	Mp	Mp	Am	Mp	Am		Mp	N			Mp	Mp	Mp	Mp	Mp	Mp	Mp				N			N	Ol	Mp	10
11	+	+	+	o	+	o	+			+	+			+	+	+	+	+							+	+	11
12	o	+	+	+	+	+	+	+	+	+	+	+	o	o	+	o	o	+			+			o	o	o	12
13	o	o	+	o	+	o	o	o	o		+	o	o	o	o	o	o	o			o			o	o	o	13
14	+	+	+	+	o	o	+	+	o	+		+	+	+	+	o		+			o				+	o	14
15	o	+	+	+	o	o	+	+	o	+		+	+	+	o	+					o				o	+	15
16	+	+	+	+	+	+	+	+	+	+	+	+	+	+	+	+	+	+			o			o	o	o	16
17	o	+	+	+	+	o	+	o	o		+	+	o	o	+	o		o						o	o		17
18	o	o	o	o	o	o	o	o	o	o	o		o	o	o	o	o	o			o			o	+	o	18
19	o	+	+	+	o		+		o	+		+	+	+	o	o		+			o				o		19
20	o	+	+	+	o	o	+			+		+	+	+	o	o		+			o				o		20
21	+	+	o	+	+	o	+	o	o	+	+	+	o	+	+	o	+	o			o			o	o	o	21
22	o	o	o	o		o	o		o	+			o	o	o	o	o	o			o			+	+	o	22
23	+	+	o			o			o	+	+	+	o	+	o	+	+				+			o	+	+	23
24	+	+	o		o	o			o	+	+		o	+	+	+	+				+			o	+	+	24
25	56	59	63	64	65	65	66	69	69	70	71	74	76	76	77	81	83	85			83			71	75	77	25
26	+	o	o	o	o	+	o	o	o	+	o	o	+	o	o	o	o	o			o			+	o	o	26
27	o	o	+	o	o	o	o	o	o	o	o	o	o	o	o	o	o	o			o			o	o	o	27
28	164	163	154	160	161	176	165	153	183	167	157	167	168	164	161	165	163	168			155			168	156	161	28
29	104	64	60	70	101	72	71	52	46	68	72	86	67	97	80	89	88	89			50			51	46	54	29
30	58	57	49	54	55	68	59	48	75	60	51	60	61	58	55	59	57	61			50			61	50	55	30
31	+79	+12	+22	+30	+84	+6	+20	+8	-39	+13	+42	+43	+10	+67	+45	+51	+51	+46			0			-16	-8	-2	31
32	+	+	+	+	+	+	+	+	+	+	+	+	+	+	+	+	+	+			+			+	+	+	32
33	U	/	/	/	/	/	/	/	/	/	/	/	/	/		/	/	/			/			U	U	U	33
33	/	/	/	/	/	/	/	/	/	/	/	/	/	/		/	/	/			/			U	U	U	33
	1	2	3	4	5	6	7	8	9	10	11	12	13	14	15	16	17	18			19			20	21	22	

Clinical Data for the Individual Patients with Hypometabolism

TABLE II

	(3.) Hypometabolism following treatment of Graves' disease								4. Invalidating polyarthritis										5. Prolonged treatment in bed, or convalescence				
	23	24	25	26	27	28	29	30	31	32	33	34	35	36	37	38	39	40	41	42	43	44	
	F	F	F	F	F	F	F	F	F	F	F	F	F	F	F	F	F	F	M	F	F	F	
	33	42	31	55	39	60	45	27	31	53	31	41	57	63	67	53	59	38	22	66	17	30	
	C	C	T	C	C	C	T	C	C	C	T	C	C	C	C	C	T	C	C	C	C	C	
1	+	0	+	+	0	+	+	+	+	+	0	+	+				+		0	+	0	0	1
2	0	+		0	0		0	0	0	+	0	0			0		0		0	0	0	0	2
3	+	+	+	0	+	+	+	+	+	+	0		+	+	+	+	+		+	+	+	+	3
4	+	+	0	+	+	+	+	0	0	+	0	+		+	0		+	0	0	+		0	4
5		+	0	0	0	+	+	0	+	0	0	0			0	0			0	0	0	0	5
6	0	+	0	0	+	0	+	0	0	0	0		0	0	0	0	0	0	0	0	0	0	6
7	0	+		0		0	+	0	0		0		0	0	0	0	0	0	0	0	0	0	7
8	+	+	+	+	0	0	+	+	+	+	0	+	+	+	0	0	+	+	0	+	0	+	8
9	0	0	+	+	0		0		0	+	0	0	0	0		0	0	0	0	0		0	9
10	N	N	N	Mp	Ol	Mp	N	N	N	Mp	N	N	Mp	Mp	Mp	Mp	Mp	N		Mp	N	Gr	10
11		+		+		+	+	+	+	+	+	+	+	+	+	+	+	+	0	+	+	+	11
12	0	+		0	0	+	0		0	0	0	+	0	0	0	0	0	0	0	0	+	0	12
13	0	0		0	+		+		0	0	0		0	0	0	0	0	0	0	0	0	0	13
14	0	0	+	0	0	0	+	0	+	0	0						0	0	0	0	0	0	14
15	0	0	0	+	0	+		0	+	0	0	+					0	0	0		0	0	15
16	0	0	0	0	+	+	0	0	0	0	0		0	0	0	0	0	0	0	0	0	0	16
17	0	0	0	0	0	+	0		0	0	0		0	0	0		0	0	0	0	0	0	17
18	+	0	0	0	+	0	0	0	0	0	0	0	0	0	0	0	0	0	0	0	0	0	18
19	0	0	0	0	0	+		0	0	0	0						0	0	0		0	0	19
20	0	0	0	0	0	+		0	0	0	0						0	0	0		0	0	20
21	0	0	0	0	0	+	0	0	0	0	0	0	0	0	0	0	0	0	0	0	0	0	21
22	0	+	+	+	+	0	0	0	0	0	0		0	0	0		0	0	0	0	+	0	22
23	0	+	+	+	0	+	+	+	0	+	0	+	+	+	+	+	+	+	0	+	0	0	23
24	+	+		+	0	+	+		0	+	0	+	+	+	+	0	+	+	0	+	0	+	24
25	78	78	82	82	83	84	85	85	75	77	82	83	83	83	84	85	86	86	62	70	72	76	25
26	0	0	0	0	0	0	0	0	+	+	0	0	0	0	0	0	0	0	+	0	0	0	26
27	0	0	0	0	0	0	0	0	0	0	0	0	0	0	0	0	0	0	+	0	0	0	27
28	150	151	168	170	161	162	164	167	159	163	153	166	167	163	150	149	154	160	175	162	160	157	28
29	55	64	55	65	47	62	73	71	61	83	43	76	82	67	73	62	63	69	69	63	66	50	29
30	45	46	61	63	55	56	58	60	53	57	48	59	60	57	45	44	49	54	68	56	54	51	30
31	+22	+39	-10	+3	-15	+11	+26	+18	+15	+46	-10	+29	+37	+18	+62	+41	+28	+28	+1	+12	+22	-2	31
32	+	+	+	+	+	0	+	+	+	0	0	0	+	+	0	0	+	0	0	+	+	+	32
33	U	/	U	U	A		U	U	/				/	U			U			U	U	/	33
33	U	/	U	U	A		U	/	/				/	U			U			U	U	/	33
	23	24	25	26	27	28	29	30	31	32	33	34	35	36	37	38	39	40	41	42	43	44	

Clinical Data for the Individual Patients with Hypometabolism

TABLE III

	(5.) Prolonged treatment in bed, or convalescence									6. Organic diseases of the nervous system																	
	45	46	47	48	49	50	51			52	53	54	55	56	57	58	59	60	61	62	63	64	65	66	67	68	
	F	F	F	F	F	M	F			F	F	F	F	M	M	F	M	M	F	M	M	M	F	M	F	F	
	52	31	19	19	29	30	62			69	55	45	31	39	64	41	63	42	35	33	45	66	34	29	62	55	
	C	T	T	T	T	T	C			C	T	C	C	C	C	C	T	T	C	C	C	T	C	C	T	C	
1	+	+	0	0	0					+	0	+	0	+	+	+	0	+		+	0	0	+		0	+	1
2	0	0	0	0	0	0				0	0		0	+	0	+	0	0		0	0	0	0	0	0	0	2
3	+	+	0	0	0	+	+			+	+	+	+	+	+	+	0	0	+	+	0	+	0	+	+	+	3
4	+	0	0	0	0	0	+			0	0		0	+	+	+	+	0		+	+	+	0		+	0	4
5	+	0	0	0	0		+			0	0		0	+	0	+	0	+			0	0	0		0	+	5
6	0	0	0	0	0	0				0	0	0	0	0	0	0	+	+	0	0	0	0	+		0	0	6
7	0		0	0	0	0	0			0	0	+	0	0	+	0	0	0	0	0	0	0	0	+	0	0	7
8	0	+	0	0	0	0	+			+	0	+	+	0	0	0	0	+	+	0	0	0	+	+	+	0	8
9	0	0	0	0	0		0			0	0		0	0	0	0	0	0	0	0	0	0	0	0	0	0	9
10	Mp	N		N	N		Mp			Mp	Mp	N	N			N			N				N		Mp	Mp	10
11		0	0	+	0	0	+			+	+	+	+	+	+	0		+	+	+	+	+	0	+	+	+	11
12	0	0	0	0	0	0	+			0	+	0	0	0	0	0	+	0	0	0	0	0	0	0	0	0	12
13	0	0	0	0	0	0				0	0	0	0	0	0	0	0	+	0	0	0	0	0	0	0	0	13
14	0	0	0	0	0					0		0	0	0	+	0	+	+	0	0	0	0	0	0	0	0	14
15	+	0	0	0	0					+		0	0	0	0	0	0	0	0		0	0	0	0	+	0	15
16	0	0	0	0	0	0	0			0	0	0	0	0	0	0	0	0	0	0	0	0	0	0	0	0	16
17	0	0	0	0	0	0	0			0	0	0	0	0	0	0	+	0	0	0	0	0	0	0	0	0	17
18	0	0	0	0	0	0	0			0	0	0	0	0	0	0	0	0	0	0	0	0	0	0	0	0	18
19	0	0	0	0	0					+			0	0	0	0	0	0	0		0	0	0	0	0	0	19
20	0	0	0	0	0					+			0	0	0	0	0	0	0		0	0	0	0	0	0	20
21	0	0	0	0	0	0	0			0	+	0	0	0	0	0	0	0	0	0	0	0	0	0	0	0	21
22	0	0	0	0	0	0	0			0		+	0	0	0	+	0	0	0		0	0	0	0	0	0	22
23	+	+	0	0	+	0	+			+	+	+	0	0	0	+	0	0	+		0	0	0	+	+	+	23
24	0	0	0	0	0	0	+			+	+	+	+	0	0	+	0	0	+	0	0	+	0	0	+	+	24
25	83	84	84	85	86	87	88			79	80	81	81	82	82	84	84	84	84	85	85	86	86	88	88	88	25
26	0	0	+	0	0	0	0			0	0	0	0	0	0	0	0	0	0	0	0	0	0	0	0	0	26
27	0	0	0	0	0	0	0			0	0	0	0	0	0	0	0	0	0	0	0	0	0	0	0	0	27
28	165	160	168	172	172	169	148			152	153	168	157	176	166	156	178	170	154	176	166	164	156	177	151	150	28
29	88	64	52	60	65	54	50			67	64	76	43	63	71	66	73	63	53	74	75	68	53	80	70	66	29
30	59	54	61	65	65	62	43			47	48	61	51	68	59	50	70	63	49	68	59	58	50	69	46	45	30
31	+49	+19	-15	-8	0	-13	+16			+43	+33	+25	-16	-7	+20	+32	+4	0	+8	+9	+27	+17	+6	+16	+52	+47	31
32	0	0	0	0	0	0	0			+	+	0	0	0	0	0	0	+	0	0	0	0	0	0	0	0	32
33										U	U							*									33
33										U	U							*									33
	45	46	47	48	49	50	51			52	53	54	55	56	57	58	59	60	61	62	63	64	65	66	67	68	

Clinical Data for the Individual Patients with Hypometabolism

TABLE IV

	(6.) Organic diseases of the nervous system			7. Chronic intoxication caused by morphine preparations or barbiturates							8. Loss of weight, and subnutrition																
	69			70	71	72	73	74			75	76	77	78	79	80	81	82	83	84	85	86	87	88	89	90	
	F			F	F	F	F	F			F	F	F	F	M	F	F	M	F	F	M	F	M	F	M	M	
	39			60	53	32	48	23			30	30	30	27	37	41	25	22	57	16	19	56	19	35	45	38	
	C			C	T	T	C	C			T	T	T	C	C	C	C	C	T	T	T	T	C	C	T	T	
1	+			+	+	0	+	0			0	+		+		0			+	+		+		+	0	+	1
2	0			0		0		0			0			0		0	0		+	0		0		0			2
3	0			+	+	+	+	+			+	+	+	+	+	+	+		+	0	0	0		+	0	+	3
4	0			+	+			0			0	+		0					+	0		0	0	0			4
5	0			+				0			0			0		0			0	0		0		0			5
6	0			+		0	+	+			0	0	0		0	+			0	0		0	0	0	0	+	6
7	0			0	+		0	0			+	+	+	0	+	0	+	+	0	0	0	0	+	+	+	0	7
8	+			+	+	+	+	0			+	+	+	0	0	+	+	0	+	0	+	+	0	+	0	+	8
9	0			0	0		0	0			0			0	0	0	0		0	0			0	0	0	0	9
10				Mp	Mp	N	Mp	N			N	N	N	N		N	N		Mp	N		Mp		N			10
11	+			+	+		+	0			+	+	+	0	+	0		+	+	0	0	+	0	+		0	11
12	0			0	0		0	+			0	+	0	0	0	0	0	0	0	0	0	0	0	0	0	0	12
13	0			0	0	0	+	+			0		0	0	0	0	0	0	0	0	0	0	0	0	0	0	13
14	0			+		0		0			0	0		0		0	0		0	0	0	+	0	0		0	14
15	0			0		0		0						0		0			+	0	0			0		0	15
16	0			0	0		0	0			0	0	0	0	0	0	0	0	0	0	0	0	0	0	0	0	16
17	0			0			0	0			0	0	0	0		0	0		0	0			0	0	0	0	17
18	0			0	0	0	0	0			0	0	0	+	0	0	0	0	0	+	0	0	0	0	0	0	18
19	0			+							0	0				0			0	0	0			0		0	19
20	0										0	0	0	0		0			+	0	0			0		0	20
21	0			0	0	0	0	0			0	0	0	0	0	0	0	0	0	0	0	0	0	0	0	0	21
22	0			0	0	0	0	0			0		0	0	0	0	0	0	+	0	0	0	0	0	0	0	22
23	+			+		0	+	0			0	+	+	0	0	0	0		+	0	0	+	0	0		0	23
24	+			+	+	0	+	0			0	+	+	0	0	0	0		+	0	0	+	0	+		0	24
25	88			73	80	84	87	88			60	75	76	78	79	80	81	82	82	83	84	84	85	85	86	86	25
26	0			0	0	0	0	0			0	0	0	0	0	0	0	+	0	0	0	0	0	0	0	0	26
27	0			0	0	0	0	0			0	0	0	0	+	0	0	0	0	0	0	0	0	0	0	0	27
28	154			168	157	159	161	162			161	161	165	161	174	159	160	175	158	163	182	159	176	162	180	174	28
29	61			62	60	51	63	55			37	46	42	50	56	44	47	67	78	48	59	110	56	43	78	62	29
30	49			61	51	53	55	56			55	55	59	55	67	53	54	68	52	57	74	53	68	56	72	67	30
31	+25			+2	+18	-4	+15	-2			-33	-16	-29	-9	-16	-17	-13	-2	+50	-16	-20	+107	-18	-23	+8	-8	31
32	0			0	+	0	0	0			0	+	+	0	0	0	0	0	+	0	0	0	0	0	0	0	32
33					U							U	U						U								33
33					U							U	/						U								
	69			70	71	72	73	74			75	76	77	78	79	80	81	82	83	84	85	86	87	88	89	90	

Clinical Data for the Individual Patients with Hypometabolism

TABLE V

	(8.) Loss of weight, and subnutrition						9. Nervous anorexia													10. Vomiting due to organic diseases			
	91	92	93	94	95	96	97	98	99	100	101	102	103	104	105	106	107	108	109	110	111	112	
	F	M	M	F	F	F	M	F	F	M	F	F	F	F	F	F	F	F	F	F	F	F	
	45	47	16	54	51	68	46	31	18	19	32	24	18	25	22	25	23	31	28	30	27	34	
	C	T	T	T	T	T	C	C	C	C	C	C	C	C	C	T	C	T	T	C	C	C	
1				+	+	0	+	+	+	0	+	0		0		+	+	+	0	+		+	1
2				0	0	0	0	+	+	0	+	0	0				0	0	0	0	0		2
3	+	+	+	+	+	0	+	+	0	0	+	+	+	+	+	+	+	+	+	+	+	+	3
4		+	0	+	0	+	0	0	0	0	+	0		0	0	0	0	0	0		0		4
5		0		0	0	0	0		0	0	0	0		0	0		0		0				5
6		+		+	0	0	0	+	+	+	0	0	+	0	0	0	0			0	0		6
7	0	0	+	+	0	+	0	0	0	+	+		+	+	+	+		0	+	+	+	+	7
8	+	+	0	+	+	+	0	0	+	+	+	0	+	0	0	+	+	+	+	+	0	+	8
9	0		0	0	0	0	0	0	0	0	0		0	0		0	0	0	0	0	0		9
10	N			Mp	Mp	Mp		N	Am		N	N	N	N	N	N	N	N	N	N	N	Gr	10
11		0		+	+	0	+			0	0	+	0	0	0	+	+	+	+	0			11
12	0	0	0	0	0	0	0	0	+	+	0	0	+	0		0	0	0	0	0	0		12
13	0	+	0	0	0	0	0		+	0	0	0	+	0		0	0	+	0	0	0		13
14		+	0	0	0	0		+	0	0	0	0	0	0	0	0	0	0	0	0	0	0	14
15		0	0	0	0	0	0		0	0	0	0	0	0	0	0	0	0	0	0	0	0	15
16	0	0	0	0	0	0	0	0	0	0	0	0	0	0	0		0	0	0	0	0	0	16
17	0	0	0	0	0	0	0	0	0	0	0	0	0	0			0	0	0		0		17
18	0	0	0	0		0	0	0	0	0	0	0	0	0	0	0	0	0	0	0	0	0	18
19			0	0	0	0	0		+	0	0	0	0	0	0	0	0	0	0	0	0	0	19
20			0	0	0	0	0		0	0	0	0	0	0	0	0	0	0	0	0	0	0	20
21	0	0	0	0	+	0	0	0	0	0	0	0	0	0	0	0	0	0	0	0	0	0	21
22	0	0	0	0	0	0	0		0	0	0	0	0	0	0	0	0	0	0	0	0		22
23	+	0	0	+	+	0	+		0	0	0		0	0	0	+	0	0	+	0	0	0	23
24		0	0	0	+	0	0	+	0	0	0	+	0	0	0	+	+	+	+	0	0	0	24
25	86	87	87	88	88	88	69	69	71	73	76	80	81	81	84	84	85	87	87	77	80	82	25
26	0	0	0	0	0	+	+	0	0	+	0	0	0	0	0	0	0	0	0	+	0	0	26
27	0	0	0	0	0	0	0	0	0	0	0	0	0	0	0	0	0	0	0	0	0	0	27
28	165	179	179	170	165	161	178	164	157	177	163	167	163	163	170	168	167	169	167	161	159	166	28
29	86	93	66	74	90	42	60	41	35	69	50	50	52	48	60	49	49	45	65	55	53	69	29
30	59	71	71	63	59	55	70	49	61	69	57	60	57	57	63	57	60	53	60	55	53	59	30
31	+46	+31	-7	+18	+53	-24	-14	-16	-32	0	-12	-17	-9	-15	-5	-14	-18	-15	+8	0	0	+15	31
32	+	0	0	+	0	0	0	0	0	0	0	0	+	0	0	0	0	0	0	0	0	0	32
33	U			U									U										33
33	A			A									U										33
	91	92	93	94	95	96	97	98	99	100	101	102	103	104	105	106	107	108	109	110	111	112	

Clinical Data for the Individual Patients with Hypometabolism

TABLE VI

	(10.) Vomiting due to organic diseases			11. Vegetarian diet through several years				12. Hypogonadism																			
	113			114	115			116	117	118	119	120	121	122	123	124	125	126	127	128	129	130	131	132	133	134	
	M			F	F			F	F	F	F	F	F	F	F	F	F	F	F	F	F	F	F	F	F	F	
	22			30	56			30	42	16	31	50	23	49	42	45	54	47	53	25	55	49	42	16	28	40	
	C			C	T			C	C	C	C	C	C	C	T	C	C	T	T	C	T	C	C	C	T	C	
1	0			0				+	+	0	+	0	+	+		+	+	+	+	+	+	0	+	+	+	+	1
2	0							+	0	0	+	0	0	0		0	0			0	0	0	0	0	+		2
3	0			+	+			+	+	+	+	+	+		+	0	+	+	+	+	+	+	+	+	+	+	3
4	0			0				+	+	0	+	+	+	+		+	0	+	+	+	+		+	0	+	+	4
5	0							0	+	0	+	+	0		0	0	0		+	0	0	0		+	+		5
6	0			0				0	+	0	0	+	+		+	0	0		0	0	0	0		+	0	+	6
7	+				+			+	+	+	0		0	0	0	0	0	0	0	+	+	+	+	0	+	+	7
8	0			+	+			+	+	0	+	+	+	+	+	0	+	+	+	+	+	+	+	+	+	0	8
9	0				0			0	0	0	0	0	0	0	0	0	0	0		0	0	0	0	0	+		9
10				Ol	Mp			N	N	Ol	Ol	Mp	Ol	Mp	Mp	Ol	Mp	Mp	Am	Ol	Mp	Mp	Ol	Ol	N	N	10
11				+	+			+	+	+	+	+	+	+		+			+	0	+	+	+	+	+	+	11
12	0			0	0			0	0	0	0	+	0	0		0	0	+	0	+	0			+	0	+	12
13	0			0	0			0	0	0	0	+	+	0	+	0	0	0	0	0	0			0	0	0	13
14	0			0				+	0	0	0	0	0			0		0		0	0	0	0	0	+		14
15	0			0				0	+	0	0	+	+			+		+		0	+	+	+	0	0	+	15
16	0			0	0			0	0	0	0	0	0	0	0	0	0	0	0	0	0	0	0	0	0	0	16
17	0			+	0			0	0	0	0	0	0	0	0	0	0	0	0	0	0	0		0	0	0	17
18	0			0	0			0	0	0	0	0	+	0	0	0	0	0	0	0	0	0	0	0	+	0	18
19	0			0				0	+	0	0		+			0		+	0	0	0			0	0		19
20	0			0				0	+	0	0		+			0		0		0	0			0	0		20
21	0			0	0			0	0	0	0	0	0	0	0	0	0	0	0	0	0	0	0	0	0	0	21
22	0			0	0			0	0	0	0	0	+		0	0	0	0	0	0	0	0		+	+		22
23				+	+			+	+	+	+	+	0		0	+		0	+	0	+	+	+	0	0	+	23
24				+	+			+	+	+	+	+	0	0	0	+	+		+	0	0	+	+	0	0	+	24
25	85			74	84			66	68	72	73	73	75	75	75	75	75	76	76	77	77	77	77	77	77	78	25
26	0			+	0			0	0	0	0	+	+	+	0	0	0	0	0	+	0	+	0	0	0	0	26
27	0			0	0			0	0	0	0	0	0	0	0	0	0	0	0	+	0	0	0	0	0	0	27
28	172			159	156			157	154	162	156	156	162	161	166	163	163	148	158	151	152	160	164	153	162	148	28
29	75			63	53			48	66	68	85	70	72	80	57	68	45	50	79	42	45	77	43	55	60	74	29
30	65			53	50			51	49	56	50	50	56	55	59	57	57	43	52	46	47	54	58	48	56	43	30
31	+15			+19	+6			-6	+35	+21	+70	+40	+29	+46	-3	+20	-21	+16	+52	-9	-4	+43	-26	+14	+7	+72	31
32	0			+	0			+	+	+	+	+	+	+	0	0	+	+	+	0	0	+	+	+	+	+	32
33				U				U	U	U	/	U	U	/			/	U	U			U	U	/	/	U	33
33				/				U	A	U	/	A	U	/			/	U	U			U	U	U	/	A	33
	113			114	115			116	117	118	119	120	121	122	123	124	125	126	127	128	129	130	131	132	133	134	

Clinical Data for the Individual Patients with Hypometabolism

TABLE VII

(12.) Hypogonadism

	135	136	137	138	139	140	141	142	143	144	145	146	147	148	149	150	151	152	153	154	155	156	157	158	159	160	
	F	F	F	F	F	F	F	F	F	F	F	F	F	F	F	F	F	F	F	F	F	F	F	F	F	F	
	58	21	45	28	26	31	16	24	21	17	16	35	47	49	55	52	52	46	16	59	49	40	45	17	22	27	
	T	C	C	T	C	T	T	T	C	T	C	C	T	C	C	C	T	C	T	C	C	C	C	C	C	C	
1	o	+	+	+	+	o	+	+	+	+	+	+	o	+	+	+	+	o	+	+	+	+	+	+	+	o	1
2	o		o	+	o		o	o		o		+	o				o	o	+	o		o	+		o		2
3	+	+	+	+	+	o	+	+	+	+	+	+	+	+	+	+	+	+	+	+	+	+	+			+	3
4	+		+		o	o	o		o	o		+	+		+	+		o	o	+		o	+	o	o	o	4
5	o	+		o	o	o	o	o		o	+	+	o				o	o	+	o	o	o	o			o	5
6	+	o			+		+	o	o	o	o	+	+		o	+	+	o	+	o		o	o		o	o	6
7	o	o	o	o	+	o	+	+	+	o	o	o	+	+	o		+	+	o	+	+	+	+		+	+	7
8	+	+	+	o	+	o	o	+	o	o	o	+	o	+	o	+	+	+	+	+	+	+	+	o	+	+	8
9		o		+	o		o	o		o	o	o	o	o	o	+	o	o	o	o	o	o	o	o	o	o	9
10	Mp	Ol	Ol	N	Ol	N	Ol	N	N	Am	Ol	N	N	N	Mp	Mp	Mp	Mp	N	Am	Mp	N	N	Am	Ol	Am	10
11	+	o	+	o	+	o	+	+		o	o	+	+	+	+	+	+	+	o	+	+	+	+		o	+	11
12	+	+	o	o	o	o	o	o	+	o	+	o	o		o	o	o	o	o	o	o	o	o	o	o	o	12
13	o	o	o	o	o		+	o	o	o	o	o	+		o	+	o	o	o	o	o	o	o	o	o	o	13
14		o			o	o	o	o	o	o	o	o		+	+	o	o	o	o	o	o	o	o	o	o	+	14
15		+			o	o	o	o	+	o	o	+		+	+	+	o	o	o	+	o	o	+	o	o	o	15
16	o	[illegible]	o	o	o		o	o	o	o	o	o		o	o	o	o	o	o	o	o	o	o	o	o	o	16
17	o	o	o		o	o	o	o		o		o		o		o	o	o	o	o	o	o	o	o	o	o	17
18	o	o	o	o	o	o	o	+	o	o	o	o	+	o	o	o	o	o	o	o	o	o	o	o	o	o	18
19	o	o			o	o	o	o		o	o	o			o		o	o	o	+		o	o		o		19
20	o	o			o	o	o	o		+	o	o			o		o	o	'o	+		o	o		o	o	20
21	o	o	o	o	o	o	o	o	o	o	+	o	o	o	o	o	o	o	o	o	o	o	o	o	o	o	21
22		+		+	o	o	+	o	+	+	+	+	o	o	o		o	o	o	o		o	+	o	+		22
23	+	+	+	+	o	+	+	+	+	o	+	+	+	+	+	+	+	o	o	o	+	+	+	o	+	o	23
24	+	o	+	+	+	o	+	o	+	o		o	+	+	+	+	o	+	o	o	+	+	+	o	o	+	24
25	78	79	79	79	79	79	79	79	80	81	81	81	81	81	81	81	82	83	83	83	83	83	83	84	84	84	25
26	o	+	o	o	o	o	o	o	o	o	o	o	o	o	+	o	o	o	o	o	o	o	o	o	o	+	26
27	o	o	o	o	o	o	o	o	o	o	o	o	o	o	o	o	o	o	o	o	o	o	o	+	o	+	27
28	160	164	164	158	164	163	160	161	159	168	163	162	148	155	165	165	167	167	174	156	159	143	155	157	165	158	28
29	85	72	67	82	56	83	51	50	62	53	73	62	67	61	105	60	79	55	69	52	61	40	63	39	56	48	29
30	54	58	58	52	58	57	64	55	53	61	57	56	43	50	69	59	60	60	67	50	53	38	50	51	59	52	30
31	+57	+24	+15	+58	-3	+46	-6	-9	+17	-13	+38	+11	+56	+22	+78	+2	+32	-8	+3	+4	+15	+5	+26	+24	-5	-10	31
32	+	+	+	+	o	o	o	o	+	+	+	+	+	+	+	+	+	o	o	o	+	o	+	o	+	+	32
33	U	U	U	U					U	U	U	U	U	U	U	U	U				U		/		/	U	33
33	U	U	U	/					A	U	U	/	A	U	U	U	A				A		U		/	U	33
	135	136	137	138	139	140	141	142	143	144	145	146	147	148	149	150	151	152	153	154	155	156	157	158	159	160	

Clinical Data for the Individual Patients with Hypometabolism

TABLE VIII

	(12.) Hypogonadism																					13. Psychoses, and severe mental depressions					
	161	162	163	164	165	166	167	168	169	170	171	172	173	174	175	176	177	178	179			180	181	182	183	184	
	F	F	F	F	F	F	F	F	F	F	F	F	F	F	F	F	F	F	F			M	F	F	F	M	
	27	56	17	23	34	51	45	50	50	39	22	45	30	42	37	45	35	53	26			45	27	27	52	22	
	T	C	C	C	T	T	C	C	C	C	C	T	T	C	T	T	C	C	T			T	C	T	C	C	
1	+		0	+	+		+	+		+		+	+	+	+	+	+		+			+		+		0	1
2			0	0	0	0		0	0	+					+	0		0	0					0		0	2
3	+	+	+	0	+	+	+	+	0	0	+	+	+	+	+	+	+	+	+			+	+	+	+	0	3
4	+	0	0	0	0			+		0		+	+	0	+	+			+			+		+	+	0	4
5		0	0		0			+		0			+	0	+	0			+				+	+		0	5
6		0	0	0	0	+	+	0	0	0	0			0	+	0		+	0			+	+	+	+	0	6
7	0		0	+	+	0	0		0	+	0	0	0	0	+	+	+	0	+			0	0	0	0	0	7
8	+	+	+	+	0	0	0	0	0	+	+	+	+	+	+	+	+	0	+			+	0	+	+	0	8
9		+	0		0			0	0	0		0			+	0		0	0			0		0		0	9
10	N	Mp	Am	Ol	Ol	Mp	Mp	Mp	Mp	Ol	Ol	N	Ol	Ol	N	Mp	Ol	Mp	N				Ol	N	Mp		10
11	+	+	0		+	+		+	+	+		+	+	+	+	+	+	+				0		+		0	11
12		0	0	+	0	0	0	0	0	0	0	0	0	0	0	0	0	0	0			+	+	0	0	0	12
13			+	0	0	+	+	0	0	0	0	0	0	0	+	0	0	0	0			+	+	+	0	0	13
14	+		0	0	0			0	0	0	0	0	0	0	0	0	0	0	0					0	0	0	14
15			0	0	0			+		0	+			+	0	+	0	0	0					+		0	15
16	0	0	0	0	0	0	0	0	0	0	0	0	0	0	0	0	0	0	0			0	0	0	0	0	16
17	0	0	0	0	0	+	0	0	0	0	0	+	0	0	0	0	0	0	0			0		0		0	17
18	0	0	0	0	0	0	+	0	0	0	+	0	0	0	0	0	0	0				0	+	0	0	0	18
19			+	0				0		0	0	0	0	+	0	0			0					0	+	0	19
20			+	0				+		0	+		0	+	0	0			0					0	+	0	20
21	0	0	0	0	0	0	0	0	0	0	0	0	0	0	0	0	+	0	0			0	0	0	0	0	21
22		0	0	+		0	+	+		0	0		+	0	0	0		0	0				0	0	0	0	22
23	+	+	0	0	+	+	0	+	+	0	0	+	+	+	+	+	+	+	0			0		0		0	23
24		+	+	0	+	+	0	+	+	+	0	+	+	+	+	+	+	+	0			0		+		0	24
25	85	85	85	85	86	86	86	87	87	87	87	87	87	87	87	88	88	88	88			72	73	75	77	78	25
26	0	0	0	+	0	0	0	0	0	0	+	0	0	0	0	0	0	+	0			+	0	0	0	+	26
27	0	0	0	0	0	0	0	0	0	0	0	0	0	0	0	0	0	0	0			0	0	0	0	+	27
28	162	151	156	157	156	164	162	164	155	156	154	157	159	162	158	161	158	154	175			176	170	156	166	172	28
29	73	104	32	61	53	62	54	73	65	48	51	61	62	50	58	44	55	71	51			75	51	49	61	65	29
30	56	46	50	51	50	58	56	58	50	50	49	51	53	56	52	55	52	49	68			68	63	50	59	65	30
31	+30	+126	-36	+20	+6	+7	-4	+26	+30	-4	+4	+20	+17	-9	+12	-20	+6	+45	-25			+10	-19	-2	+3	0	31
32	+	+	0	+	0	0	+	+	0	0	+	+	0	0	+	0	+	+	0			+	0	0	0	0	32
33	U	U		U			U	U			U	/			U		U	/				U					33
33	U	/		/			/	/			U	U			U		U	/				/					33
	161	162	163	164	165	166	167	168	169	170	171	172	173	174	175	176	177	178	179			180	181	182	183	184	

Clinical Data for the Individual Patients with Hypometabolism

TABLE IX

	(13.) Psychoses, and severe mental depressions										14. Sclerodermia	15. Amputations of extremities				16. Uncertain cases of hypometabolism					
	185	186	187	188	189	190	191	192	193	194	195	196	197	198	199	200	201	202	203	204	
	F	M	M	F	M	F	F	M	F	F	F	F	F	F	F	F	F	F	M	F	
	37	33	39	26	43	26	17	35	66	32	17	67	47	49	42	19	49	44	25	24	
	C	C	C	T	C	T	C	T	T	C	C	C	T	C	C	C	C	C	C	C	
1	+	o	o	o	o	o	o	+	o		+	o			+	+	+	o	+	+	1
2	+	o	o	o	o			o	o			o	o			o	o		o	+	2
3	+	+	+	+	o	+	+	o	+	+	o	+	+	+	+	+	+	+	+	+	3
4	+	o	+	+	o	o		o		+	o	o	o		o	o	+		o	+	4
5	+	o	o		o			o	+		o	o	o	+		+			o	+	5
6	+	+	+	+	o	+	+	+		+	o	o	o	+	o	o			o	+	6
7	o	o	o	o	+	o	o	o	+	o	o	o	o	o	+	o	+		o	o	7
8	+	o	o	+	o	+	o	o	+	o	o	o	o	o	+	+	+	+		o	8
9	o	o	o	o	o	o	o	o		o	o	o	o	o	+	o	o	o		o	9
10	N			N		Gr	Ol		Mp	N	N	Mp	Mp	Mp	N	N	Mp	N		Am	10
11	+	+	o			o		+	o	o	o	+	+	+	+		+	+		o	11
12	+	o	o		o	o	+	o	+	+	o	o	o	o	+	o	+	o	+	+	12
13	+	+	+	+	o	+	+	+	+	+	o	o	o	o	o	o	+		+	+	13
14	o	o	o	o	o	o	o	o		o	o	o	o		o	o	o	o	o	o	14
15	o	o	o	o	o		o	o		o	o	o	o		o	o	o	o	+	o	15
16	o	o	o	o	o	o	o	o		o	o	o	o	o	o	o	o	o	o	o	16
17	o	o	o	o	o	o	o	o	o	o	o	o	o	o	o	o	o	o	o	o	17
18	o	o	o	o	o	o	o	o	o	o	o	o	o	o	o	o	o	o	o	o	18
19	o	o	o	o	o		o	o		o	o	o		o	o	o	o	o	o	o	19
20	o	o	o		o	o	o	o		o	o	o	+		o	o	o	o	o	o	20
21	o	o	o	o	o	o	o	o	o	o	o	o	o	o	o	o	o	o	o	o	21
22	+	o	o	o	o	o	+	o	o	o	+	o	+		o	+		o	o	+	22
23	+	+	o	o	o	o	+	o	+	o	o	+	+	+	+	o	+	o	o	o	23
24	+	+	o	+	o	o	o	o	+	o	o	+	+	+	+	o	+		o	o	24
25	79	82	82	82	83	85	85	85	88	88	78	81	87	87	87	63	65	70	70	71	25
26	o	o	+	o	+	o	o	o	o	o	+	o	o	o	o	+	o	o	o	o	26
27	o	o	o	o	o	o	o	o	o	o	o	o	o	o	o	o	o	o	o	o	27
28	163	173	171	170	175	156	154	183	152	170	166	173	153	152	155	167	169	155	172	168	28
29	59	89	72	64	67	59	55	60	47	63	58	99	63	61	56	81	55	76	66	57	29
30	57	66	64	63	68	50	49	75	47	63	59	66	48	47	50	60	62	50	65	61	30
31	+4	+36	+13	+2	-1	+18	+12	-20	0	0	-2					+35	-11	+52	+2	-7	31
32	+	+	o	o	o	o	+	o	o	o	o					+	+	+	o	+	32
33	*	U					U									U	U	/		U	33
33	*	U					A									/	U	U		/	33
	185	186	187	188	189	190	191	192	193	194	195	196	197	198	199	200	201	202	203	204	

Clinical Data for the Individual Patients with Hypometabolism

TABLE X

(16.) Uncertain cases of hypometabolism

	205	206	207	208	209	210	211	212	213	214	215	216	217	218	219	220	221	222	223	224	225	226	227	228	229	230	
	F	M	M	F	F	M	F	M	M	F	F	F	F	M	M	M	F	F	F	F	M	F	F	F	F	F	
	34	23	32	20	67	45	23	34	44	41	19	55	59	46	41	24	23	52	28	28	34	56	20	23	23	20	
	T	T	C	C	C	C	T	C	T	T	T	T	T	T	C	C	C	C	T	C	C	C	T	C	T	C	
1	+	+	0	+	+	0	0	+	0	+	+	+	+	+	+	0	0		+	+	0	+		+		+	1
2	0	0	0		0	+	0	0	0	+	0	+		0	+	0	0				0	0				0	2
3	+	+	+	+	+	+	+	0	0	+	+	+	+	+	0	0	0	+	+	+	0	+			+	+	3
4	0	+		0	+	0	0	+	0	+	0	+	0	+	0	0	0	+	+		0	+		0		0	4
5	+	+		+	0	+	0	0	0	0	+	+		+	0	0	0	0		+	0	0	0			0	5
6	0	0			0	0	0	0	0	+	0	+	0	0	0	0	0	0	0		0	0	0		0	0	6
7	0	+	0	+	0	0	0	0	0	+	0	+	+	+	0	+	0	+	0	+	0	0	0	0		0	7
8	0	0	0	0	+	0	0	0	0	+	0	+	+	+	0	0	+	+	+	0	0	+	+	+	0	0	8
9	0	0	0	0	0		0	0	0	+	0	+	0	0	0	+	0	0		0	0	0	0	0	+	0	9
10	N			N	Mp		N			N	Ol	Mp	Mp				N	Mp	N	N		Mp	N	N	N	N	10
11			+		+	+	0		+	+	0	+	+	+	+	0	0	+	+		+	+			+	+	11
12	0	0	0	0	0	0	0	0	0	0	0	0	0	0	0	0	0	+	0		0	0	0	0	0	0	12
13	0	0	0	0	0	0	0	0	0	+	0	0	0	0	0	0	0	0	0		0	0	0		0	0	13
14	0	0	0	0	0	0	0	+		+	0	+	0	+	+	0	0		0	0	0	0	0	0	0	0	14
15	0	0	0	0	0	0	0	0	0	0		+	0	+	+	0	0		0	0	0	0	0	+	0	0	15
16	0	0	0	0	0	0	0	0	0	0	0	0	0	0	0	0	0	0	0	0	0	0	0		0	0	16
17	0	0		0	0	0	0	0	0	0	0	0	0	0	0	0	0	0	0	0	0	0				0	17
18	0	0	0	0	0	0	0	0	0	0	0	0	0	0	0	0	0	0	0	0	0	0	0	0	0	0	18
19	0	0	0	0	0	0	0	0	0	0		+	0	0	0	0	0			0		0	0	0	0	0	19
20	0	0	0	0	0	0	0	0	0	0		+	0	0	0	0	0			0	0	0	0	+	0	0	20
21	0	0	0	0	0	0	0	0	0	0	0	0	0	0	0	0	0	0	0	0	0	0	0		0	0	21
22	0	0	0	0	0	0	0	0	0	0	0	0		0	0	0	0	0	0	+	0	0	0	+		0	22
23	0	0	+		+	0	0	0	0	+		+	+		0	0	0	+	+	+	0	+			+	0	23
24	0	0	+	0	+	+	0	0	+	+		+	+	+	+	0	0	+	+	0	+	+			+	+	24
25	71	72	72	72	72	73	74	75	75	75	76	76	76	76	76	76	77	77	77	77	78	79	79	79	79	79	25
26	+	+	+	0	0	0	0	0	0	+	+	+	0	+	0	0	+	0	0	0	0	0	0	+	0	0	26
27	0	0	0	0	0	0	0	0	0	0	0	0	0	0	0	0	0	0	0	0	0	0	0	0	0	0	27
28	166	170	174	160	157	186	165	184	175	158	164	160	164	176	170	170	151	164	174	152	175	162	159	165	162	155	28
29	68	66	65	51	62	85	64	84	100	76	53	79	57	70	71	61	56	60	87	50	67	69	57	67	60	52	29
30	59	63	67	54	51	77	59	76	68	52	58	54	58	68	63	63	46	58	67	47	68	56	53	59	56	50	30
31	+15	+5	-3	-6	+22	+10	+9	+11	+47	+46	-9	+46	-2	+3	+13	-3	+22	+4	+30	+6	-1	+23	+8	+14	+7	+4	31
32	0	0	+	+	+	0	0	+	0	+	0	+	+	+	+	0	+	+	+	+	0	+	+	+	0	0	32
33			I	I	I			U		U		U	U	I	U		U	U	U	*		U	U	U			33
33			U	U	I			U		A		I	A	U	I		U	U	U	*		U	U	U			33
	205	206	207	208	209	210	211	212	213	214	215	216	217	218	219	220	221	222	223	224	225	226	227	228	229	230	

TABLE XI

(16.) Uncertain cases of hypometabolism.

	231	232	233	234	235	236	237	238	239	240	241	242	243	244	245	246	247	248	249	250	251	252	253	254	255	256	
	F	M	F	F	F	F	F	M	F	F	M	F	M	F	F	F	F	F	F	F	M	F	M	F	M	F	
	18	29	20	37	21	27	39	59	19	18	55	58	35	30	26	46	44	66	18	17	57	41	22	17	27	18	
	C	C	C	C	C	T	C	T	C	C	C	T	C	C	T	T	C	T	C	C	C	C	C	C	T	C	
1	+	0	+	0	+	+	+	0	0		+	0	0	+	+		+	0	+	0		+	0	+	+	0	1
2	0	+			0	+		0	0		0		0	+	0		+	0	+	0	0	+	0	0	0	0	2
3	+	0	+	0	+	+	+	0	0			+	+	+	+	+	+	+	+	0	+	+	0	+	+	+	3
4	+	0		0	0	0		0	0		+	+	0	+	0		0	0	0	0	+	+	0	0	0	0	4
5	+	0		0	0	+	0	0	0		+	0	+	0	0	0	+	0	+	0		0	0	+	0	0	5
6	+	0	0	0	0	+	0	0	0	+	0	0	0	+	0		+	0	0	0	+	0	0	0	0	0	6
7		0	0	0	+	+	+	0	0	+	0	0	+	0	0	0	+	0	0	0	+	0	0	0	0	0	7
8	0	0	+	0	+	+	0	0	0	0	0	+	0	0	+	+	0	0	+	0	0	0	0	0	0	0	8
9	0	0	0	0	0	0	0	0	0	0	0	0	0	0	0		0	0		0	0	0	0	0		0	9
10	N		N	N	N	N	N			N		Mp		N	N	N	Ol	Mp	N	N		N		N		N	10
11	+	0	+	+	0	+	+	+	0	0	+	+	+	+	0	+	+	+	0	0		+	0	+			11
12	0	0	0	0	0	0	0	0	0	0	0	0	0	0	0	0	0	0	0	0	+	0	0	0	0	+	12
13	0	0	0	0	0	0	0	0	0	0	0	0	0	0	0	0	0	0	0	0	+	0	0	0	0	0	13
14	0	0	0	0	0	0	0	0	0	0	0		0	0	0	0	0	0	0	0		0	0	0	0	0	14
15	0	0	0		0	0	0	0	0		0	+	0	0	0	0	+	0	0	0	0	0	0	0	0	0	15
16	0	0	0	0	0	0	0	0	0	0	0	0	0	0	0	0	0	0	0	0	0	0	0	0	0	+	16
17	0	0	0	0	+	0		0	0		0	0	0	0	0	0	0	0	0	0	0	0	0	0	0	0	17
18	+	0	0	0	0	0	0	0	0	0	0	0	0	0	0	0	0	0	0	0	0	0	0	0	0	0	18
19	0	0		+	0	0	0	0	0		0		0	0		0	+	0	0	0		0	0	0	0	0	19
20	0	0		+	0	0	0	0	0		0		0	0		0	0	0	0	0		0	0	0	0	0	20
21	0	0	0	0	0	0	0	0	0	0	0	0	0	0	0	0	0	0	0	0	0	0	0	0	0	0	21
22	+	0	+	+	+	0	0	0	+	0	0		0	+	+	0	0	0	+	0	0	0	0	+		+	22
23	0	0	+	+	0	0	+	0	0		0	+	+	0	0	+	+	+	+	0		+	0	+	0	+	23
24	+	0	+	+	0	+	+	+	0		0	+	+	0	0	+	+	+	0	0		+	0	+	0	0	24
25	79	79	79	80	80	80	80	80	80	80	81	81	81	81	81	81	81	82	82	82	83	83	83	83	83	83	25
26	+	0	0	+	0	+	0	+	0	0	+	0	0	0	0	0	0	+	0	0		0	+	0	0	0	26
27	0	0	0	0	0	0	0	0	+	0	0	0	0	0	0	0	0	0	0	0		0	0	0	0	0	27
28	169	176	161	159	163	163	152	170	171	164	173	159	185	151	158	149	172	158	156	167	165	157	163	166	173	155	28
29	88	67	67	82	64	62	70	68	66	51	56	60	75	54	48	66	75	89	65	55	68	52	57	77	94	63	29
30	62	68	55	53	57	57	56	63	64	58	66	53	77	46	52	44	65	52	50	60	59	51	57	54	66	50	30
31	+42	-2	+22	+55	+12	+9	+25	+8	+3	-12	-15	+13	-3	+17	-8	+50	+15	+71	+30	-8	+15	+2	0	+43	+43	+26	31
32	+	0	+	0	+	+	+	0	0	0	0	0	+	+	+	+	0	0	+	0	+	0	0	+	+	+	32
33	U		/		U	/	U						U	U	/	U			U		U			U	U	U	33
33	U		/		U	/	A						U	/	/	U			U		U			/	U	U	33
	231	232	233	234	235	236	237	238	239	240	241	242	243	244	245	246	247	248	249	250	251	252	253	254	255	256	

Clinical Data for the Individual Patients with Hypometabolism

TABLE XII

(16.) Uncertain cases of hypometabolism.

	257	258	259	260	261	262	263	264	265	266	267	268	269	270	271	272	273	274	275	276	277	278	279	280	281	282	
	F	F	M	F	F	M	F	F	F	F	F	M	M	F	M	M	F	F	F	F	F	M	M	F	M	M	
	21	39	49	20	69	24	59	60	55	28	21	41	42	19	52	23	42	25	61	28	24	34	22	19	16	27	
	C	T	T	C	T	C	C	T	C	T	C	T	T	C	C	C	C	C	C	C	T	T	C	T	C	T	
1	+	o		+	+	o	+	+	+	+			o	+	o	o		+	o	+	o	o	o	+	o	o	1
2		o		o		o			o	+	+	o	o		o	o			o	o	o		o		o	o	2
3	+	o		+		o	+	+	o	+	+	+	o	+	+	+	+	+	+	o	+		+	+	o	o	3
4	o	o	o	o	+	o		+	o	+			o	o	+	o		o	o	o	o			o	o	o	4
5	+	o	o	+		o	+	o					o			o	o	o	o	o	+	o			o	o	5
6	o	o	o	o		o	+	o			o		o		+	+	o	o	o	o	+	o	+	o	o	o	6
7	o	o	o	o	o	o	o	o	o	+		o	o	o	o	o		o	o	+	o	+	+	+	o	o	7
8	+	o	o	o	o	o	+	+	+	o	+	o	o	+	o	o	+	o	o	o	o	+	o	+	o	o	8
9	o	o		o		o		o	o			o	o	o	o	o		o	o	o	o		o	o	o	o	9
10	N	N		N	Mp		Mp	Mp	Mp	N	N			N			N	N	Mp	N	N	.		N			10
11		+	+	o	+	o	+		+		+	+	o	+	+	o		o	+	o	+		+	+	+	o	11
12	o	o		o	o	o	+		o	o	o	o	o	+	o	o	o	o	o	o	o	o	o	o	o	o	12
13	o	o		o	+	o	+		o	o	+	o	o	o	+	+	o	o	o	o	o	o	+	o	o	o	13
14	o	o		o	+	o	o	+		o		o	o	o		o	o	o	o	o	o	o	o		o	o	14
15	o	+	o	o	+	o	o		+			o	o	o	o	o	o	o	o	+	o	o	o	o	o	o	15
16	o	o	o	o	o	o	o	o	o	o	o	o	o	o	o	o	o	o	o	o	o	o	o	o	o	o	16
17	o	o		o	o	o	o		o	o	o	o	o	o	o	o	o	+	o	o	o	o	o		o	o	17
18	o	o	o	o	o	o	o	o	+	+	+	o	+	o	o	+	o	+	o	o	+	o	o	o	o	o	18
19	o	o		o	o	o	o					o	o	o	o	o	o	o	o	o	o	o	o		o	o	19
20	o	o		o	+	o	o					o	o	o	o	o	o		o	o	o	o	o		o	o	20
21	o	o	o	o	o	o	o	o	o	o	o	o	o	o	o	o	o	o	o	o	o	o	o	o	o	o	21
22	o	o	o	+	o	o	o	o	o	+	+	o	o	+	o	o	o	o	o	o	o	o	o	+	o	o	22
23		+	+	o	+	o	+	+	o	o	+	o	o	+	+	o	+	o	+	o	o		o	+	o	o	23
24		+	+	o	+	o	+	+	+	o	+	+	o	+	+	o	+	o	o	o	o		+	o	o	o	24
25	83	83	83	83	84	84	84	84	84	84	84	84	84	84	84	85	85	85	85	85	85	85	86	86	86	86	25
26	o	o	o	o	o	o	o	o	o	+	o	+	o	o	+	o	o	o	o	o	o	o	+	o	+	o	26
27	o	o	o	o	o	+	o	o	o	o	o	o	o	o	o	o	o	o	o	o	o	o	o	o	o	o	27
28	162	160	176	161	152	172	157	156	162	165	164	182	182	162	176	168	162	157	163	157	156	179	168	168	174	168	28
29	56	66	85	64	71	67	75	71	81	64	52	65	77	61	71	72	101	52	70	60	52	74	65	76	65	56	29
30	56	54	68	55	47	65	51	50	56	59	58	74	74	56	68	61	56	51	57	51	50	71	61	61	67	61	30
31	0	+22	+25	+16	+50	+ 3	+47	+42	+45	+ 8	-10	-12	+ 4	+ 9	+ 4	+16	+80	+ 2	+23	+18	+ 4	+ 4	+ 7	+25	-3	-8	31
32	+	o	+	o	+	o	+	+	+	+	+	o	o	o	+	o	+	o	+	+	+	o	+	+	o	o	32
33	U		*		U		U	U	U	U	U				*		U		/	*	U		U	/			33
33	/		*		U		/	U	A	/	/				*		/		U	*	/		U	/			33
	257	258	259	260	261	262	263	264	265	266	267	268	269	270	271	272	273	274	275	276	277	278	279	280	281	282	

Clinical Data for the Individual Patients with Hypometabolism

TABLE XIII

(16.) Uncertain cases of hypometabolism

	283	284	285	286	287	288	289	290	291	292	293	294	295	296	297	298	299	300	301	302	303	304	305	306	307	308	
	M	F	F	F	F	F	F	F	M	F	F	F	F	F	M	F	F	F	F	F	F	M	F	M	F	M	
	55	16	17	31	24	36	23	55	54	58	39	30	21	59	48	31	44	21	18	27	25	31	20	21	35	36	
	C	C	C	C	C	T	T	C	T	C	C	T	T	C	T	T	C	C	C	T	T	C	C	T	C	C	
1	0	+	+	0	+	+	+	+	0		0	+	0	+	0	+	+	0	+	+		0	0	0	0	0	1
2			+	0		0			0	0			0	+	0	0		0	+	0		0	0	0	0		2
3	0	+	+	+	+	+	+	+	+	+		+	+	+		+	+	0	0	0	+	0	0	+	0	+	3
4	0	0	0	0		0	+	+	+	0	0		0	+	0	0		0	0	0	0	0	0	0	0	0	4
5	0	0	0	+	+	0	+	+	+	0			0	0	0	0		0	0	+	0	0	0	0	0	0	5
6	0		0	0	+	0	+	+	0	0	0		0	+	0	0		0		0	0	0	0	0	0	0	6
7	0	0	0	+		0	0	+	0	0	0	0	0	0	0	0	+	0	0	0	0	0	0	0	0	0	7
8	+	+	0	0	+	0	0	+	0	0	0	0	0	0	0	+	0	0	0	0	0	0	0	0	0	0	8
9	0	0	0	0	0	0	0	0	0	0	0	0	0	0		0	0	0		0	0	0	0	0	0	0	9
10		N	N	N	N	N	N	Mp		Mp	N	Ol	N	Mp		N	N	N	N	N	N		N		N		10
11	0	+	0	+		+	+	+	0	+	0		+	+	+	+	+	0	+	+	+	+	+	0	0	0	11
12	0	0	0	0		0	+	0	0	0	0	+	0	0	0	0	0	+	0	0	0	0	0	0	0	0	12
13	0	0	0	0		0	+	0	0	0	0		0	+	0	0	0	0		0	0	0	0	0	0	0	13
14		0	0	0	+	0	+	0			+	0	0	+		0	0	0	0	0	0	0	0		0	0	14
15		0	0	0				0	0		+		0	+		0		0		0	+	0	0		0		15
16	0	0	0	0		0	0	0	0	0	0		0	0	0	0	0	0	0	0	0	0	0	0		0	16
17	0	0	0	0	0	0	0	0	0		0	0	0	0	0	0	0	0	0	0	0	0	0	+	0	0	17
18	0	0	+	+	+	0	0	0	0	0	0	+	+	0	0	0	0	0	0	0	0	0	0	+	0	0	18
19		0	0	0				0	0				0	+		0	0	0	0	0	0	0	0		0		19
20		0	0	+					0		+		0	+		0	0	0	0	0	0	0	0		0		20
21	0	0	0	0	0	0	0	+	0	0	0	+	0	+	0	0	0	0	0	0	0	0	0	0	0	0	21
22	0	+	+	0		0	+	0	0	0		+	+	0	0	+	+	0	+	0	0	0	0		0	0	22
23	0	+	0	0	+		+	+	0	+	+	+	+	+	0	+	+	0	+	0	+	+	0	0	0		23
24	0	+	0	0	+	+	+	+	0	+	+	+	+	0	0	+	+	0	0	0	+	0	0	0	0		24
25	86	86	86	87	87	87	87	87	87	87	87	88	88	88	88	88	88	88	88	88	88	88	88	88	88	88	25
26	+	0	0	0	0	0	0	0	0	0	0	0	0	0	0	0	0	0	0	0	0	0	0	0	0	+	26
27	0	0	0	0	0	0	0	0	0	0	0	0	0	0	0	0	0	0	0	0	0	0	0	0	0	0	27
28	170	156	158	152	159	170	161	175	166	156	159	163	159	157	148	159	170	176	160	159	166	170	167	181	165	180	28
29	82	58	55	61	52	56	81	76	86	73	107	59	51	85	84	54	60	87	71	93	100	75	59	77	76	73	29
30	63	50	52	47	53	63	55	67	59	50	53	57	53	51	76	53	63	68	54	53	59	63	60	73	59	72	30
31	+30	+16	+6	+30	-2	-11	+47	+13	+46	+46	+102	+3	-4	+68	+11	+2	-5	+28	+31	+75	+70	+19	-2	+5	+29	+2	31
32	+	+	0	0	+	0	0	+	+	0	0	0	0	+	0	0	0	0	+	0	+	0	0	0	+	0	32
33	U	*			/			U	*					U					U		U				U		33
33	/	*			/			U	*					/					/		U				/		33
	283	284	285	286	287	288	289	290	291	292	293	294	295	296	297	298	299	300	301	302	303	304	305	306	307	308	

Case Number

Sex

Age in Years

Place of Residence

1. Chilliness
2. Decreased Sweating
3. Fatigue
4. Impairment of Memory and Reduced Power of Inculcation
5. Somnolence
6. Depression
7. Dyspepsia
8. Constipation
9. Oliguria
10. Conditions of Menstruation
11. Rheumatism
12. Apathy
13. Objectively observed Depression
14. Scantiness of the Hair of the Scalp
15. Scantiness of the Eyebrows
16. Changes in the Skin of the Face
17. Hoarseness
18. Enlargement of the Thyroid Gland
19. Scantiness of Axillary Hair
20. Scantiness of Pubic Hair
21. Thickening of the Skin and Subcutaneous Tissues of the Extremities
22. Perniosis
23. Subcutaneous Infiltrations
24. Myalgiae
25. Metabolic Rate in per cent of Normal
26. Bradycardia
27. Hypothermia
28. Height in Centimeters
29. Observed Body Weight in Kilograms
30. Ideal Body Weight in Kilograms
31. Deviation from Ideal Body Weight in per cent
32. Thyroid Administration

33 Objective Effect of Thyroid Administration

33. Subjective Effect of Thyroid Administration

Case Number

EXPLANATION OF SYMBOLS USED IN THE APPENDED TABLES

F: Female
M: Male
C: Country
T: Town
N: Normal menstruation
Am: Amenorrhoea
Gr: Gravidity
Mp: Menopause
Ol: Oligomenorrhoea
I: Improved
U: Unchanged
A: Aggravated
*: Observation period too short for estimation of effect of thyroid administration

CLINICAL NOTES

Group 1: Genuine myxedema.

1—8. Myxedema.
9. Myxedema (Josephson's variety).
10—18. Myxedema.

Group 2: Congenital myxedema.

19. Congenital Myxedema.

Group 3: Hypometabolism following treatment of Graves' disease.

20. Subtotal thyroidectomy 1926.
21. Subtotal thyroidectomy 1926.
22. Subtotal thyroidectomy 1936.
23. Thyroiditis 1920.
24. X-ray treatment of thyroid in 1918.
25. Subtotal thyroidectomy 1932.
26. Graves' disease 1910, medically treated.
27. X-ray treatment of thyroid in 1929.
28. Subtotal thyroidectomy 1925.
29. X-ray treatment of thyroid in 1921.
30. Subtotal thyroidectomy 1935.

Group 4: Invalidating polyarthritis.

31—40. Polyarthritis.

Group 5: Prolonged treatment in bed, or convalescence.

41. Convalescence following brucellosis.
42. Prolonged treatment in bed. Neurasthenia.
43. Prolonged treatment in bed following rheumatic fever.
44. Prolonged treatment in bed following influenza.
45. Prolonged treatment in bed on account of ulcer of the leg.
46. Convalescence following scarlet fever.
47. Convalescence following pleurisy.
48. Convalescence following rheumatic fever.
49. Prolonged treatment in bed on account of abscess of the lung.
50. Prolonged treatment in bed following pulmonary inflammation.
51. Prolonged treatment in bed previous to admission to hospital due to coronary sclerosis.

Group 6: Organic diseases of the nervous system.

52. Cerebral thrombosis.
53. Cerebral hemorrhage.
54. Disseminated sclerosis.
55. Arachnoiditis.
56. Disseminated sclerosis.
57. Cerebral arteriosclerosis.
58. Disseminated encephalomyelitis.
59. Cerebral thrombosis.
60. Tumor of the brain.
61. Myelopathy.
62. Disseminated sclerosis.
63. Disseminated sclerosis.
64. Cerebral arteriosclerosis.
65. Arachnoiditis.
66. Paralysis following poliomyelitis.
67. Cerebral thrombosis.
68. Disseminated sclerosis.
69. Syringomyelia.

Group 7: Chronic intoxication caused by morphine preparations or barbiturates.

70. Chronic morphine intoxication.
71. Chronic codeine intoxication.
72. Chronic barbiturate intoxication.
73. Chronic opium intoxication.
74. Chronic morphine intoxication.

Group 8: Loss of weight, and subnutrition.

75. Duodenal ulcer. Considerable loss of weight.
76. Subnutrition.
77. Subnutrition.
78. Neurasthenia. Loss of weight of 10 kg during a period of three months.
79. Subnutrition.
80. Loss of weight.
81. Dyspepsia. Reduction of weight 13 kg.
82. Gastric ulcer. Dietary treatment for one month previous to determination of basal metabolism.
83. Loss of weight on reduction diet.
84. Subnutrition.
85. Subnutrition.
86. Loss of weight on reduction diet.
87. Subnutrition.
88. Polyposis of the colon with frequent bloody stools.
89. Duodenal ulcer. Determination of basal metabolism after one month's dietary treatment and confinement to bed.
90. Neurasthenia. Reduction of weight 15 kg during a three month period.
91. Loss of weight on reduction diet.
92. Loss of weight on reduction diet.
93. Duodenal ulcer. Loss of weight following dietary treatment.
94. Dyspepsia. Reduction of weight of 15 kg during a three month period.
95. Loss of weight on reduction diet.
96. Subnutrition.

Group 9: Nervous anorexia.

97—109. Nervous anorexia.

Group 10: Vomiting due to organic diseases.

110. Gastric ulcer. Copious vomitings for several weeks before admission.
111. Diverticulum of the stomach.
112. Hyperemesis gravidarum.
113. Cholelithiasis associated with frequent vomiting.

Group 11: Vegetarian diet through several years.

114—115. Vegetarian diet through several years.

Group 12: Hypogonadism.

116. Cystic degeneration of ovaries demonstrated at operation for gonorrhoic salpingitis.
117. Irregular menstruation. Hot flushes.
118. Nearly complete amenorrhoea. Hot flushes.
119. Menstruation very sparse. Moderate mental depression.
120. Marked hot flushes and fits of profuse sweating.
121. Hot flushes and fits of sweating.
122. Ovariectomy in 1923. Climacterial symptoms since 1924.
123. Hot flushes and attacks of sweating.
124. Attacks of hot flushes.
125. Hot flushes. Fits of sweating.
126. Menopause one year previous to admission. Hot flushes.
127. Hypertrichosis of upper lip.
128. Menstruation sparse. Intervals of menstrual cycle three months.
129. Marked hot flushes and climacterial symptoms.
130. Menstruation sparse during the last four years. Marked attacks of hot flushes.
131. Hot flushes and attacks of sweating.
132. Intervals of menstrual cycle three months.
133. Amenorrhoea. Menstruation provoked through hormone treatment.
134. Attacks of hot flushes.
135. Attacks of hot flushes.
136. Menstruation sparse since puberty. Secondary amenorrhoea.
137. Marked oligomenorrhoea since puberty.
138. Marked oligomenorrhoea. Treated with estrone.
139. Ovariectomy performed 1932.
140. Menstruation irregular. Frigidity and attacks of sweating.
141. Oligomenorrhoea. Mental depression.
142. Genital hypoplasia.
143. Secondary amenorrhoea.
144. Primary amenorrhoea.
145. Secondary amenorrhoea (through a period of two years).
146. Attacks of hot flushes. Frigidity and mental depression.
147. Marked climacterial symptoms. Hot flushes and attacks of sweating.
148. Marked oligomenorrhoea. Attacks of hot flushes and sweating.
149. Attacks of hot flushes.
150. Menopause two years previous to admission.
151. Marked hot flushes and attacks of sweating.
152. Hot flushes.
153. Amenorrhoea through a period of three months.
154. Attacks of sweating.
155. Marked attacks of hot flushes.
156. Menstruation irregular and very sparse.
157. Beginning climacterial symptoms with attacks of hot flushes.

158. Amenorrhoea during a period of six months.
159. Menstruation sparse and infrequent.
160. Attacks of sweating.
161. Menstruation sparse and irregular.
162. Attacks of hot flushes.
163. Primary amenorrhoea. Retarded mental development.
164. Menstruation very sparse. Long periods of amenorrhoea.
165. Oligomenorrhoea since puberty.
166. Amenorrhoea during a period of twenty years.
167. Beginning climacterial complaints. Attacks of hot flushes.
168. Menstruation always very sparse. Menopause occurred at the age of 42.
169. Menstruation very sparse during the last ten years with intervals between menstruations up to one year.
170. Oligomenorrhoea. Intervals of menstrual cycle three to four months. Attacks of hot flushes.
171. Intervals of menstrual cycle three to four months.
172. Attacks of hot flushes.
173. Ovariectomy on right side 1937. Cystic degeneration of left ovary.
174. Menstruation irregular and sparse.
175. Oligomenorrhoea. Duration of menstrual period two days. Frigidity.
176. X-ray treatment of ovaries. Attacks of hot flushes and sweating.
177. Oligomenorrhoea through a period of several years.
178. Marked attacks of hot flushes.
179. Genital hypoplasia. Rightsided oophoritis.

Group 13: Psychoses, and severe mental depressions.

180. Psychosis.
181. Psychogenic psychosis.
182. Mental depression.
183. Posttraumatic psychosis.
184. Posttraumatic psychosis.
185. Psychosis.
186. Psychosis.
187. Psychosis of manio-depressive type.
188. Schizophrenic psychosis.
189. Psychosis of paranoid type.
190. Mental depression in pregnancy.
191. Mental depression.
192. Psychosis of manio-depressive type.
193. Psychosis of manio-depressive type.
194. Psychogenic psychosis.

Group 14: Sclerodermia.

195. Sclerodermia.

Group 15: Amputations of extremities.

196. Amputation of left leg below the knee.
197. Amputation of left leg below the knee.
198. Amputation of right leg below the knee.
199. Amputation of left foot.

Group 16: Uncertain cases of hypometabolism.

200. Obesity. Chronic constipation.
201. Coronary sclerosis. Chronic constipation. Cholelithiasis.
202. Normal.
203. Neurasthenia.

204. Neurasthenia.
205. Cholelithiasis.
206. Neurasthenia.
207. Normal.
208. Neurasthenia.
209. Coronary sclerosis.
210. Prolapse of lumbar intervertebral disc. Neurasthenia. No reduction of physical activities.
211. Normal.
212. Eczema.
213. Obesity.
214. Abdominal complaints following cholecystectomy.
215. Normal.
216. Arterial hypertension. Obesity.
217. Chronic cholecystitis. Cholelithiasis.
218. Chronic constipation.
219. Eczema.
220. Normal.
221. Posttraumatic epilepsy.
222. Valvular aortic disease.
223. Chronic constipation.
224. Neurasthenia.
225. Prolapse of lumbar intervertebral disc. No reduction of physical activities.
226. Normal.
227. Chronic constipation.
228. Chronic constipation.
229. Normal.
230. Cardiac neurosis.
231. Congenital syphilis.
232. Cardiac neurosis.
233. Lumbago.
234. Obesity.
235. Chronic constipation. Colitis.
236. Chronic constipation.
237. Myalgia.
238. Spondylitis.
239. Normal.
240. Normal.
241. Oligophrenia.
242. Neurasthenia.
243. Normal.
244. Oligophrenia.
245. Chronic constipation.
246. Neurasthenia. Myalgia. Chronic cholecystitis. Obesity.
247. Cholelithiasis.
248. Arthritis of knee joints. Obesity.
249. Cephalalgia.
250. Asthenia.
251. Cerebral arteriosclerosis.
252. Myalgia.
253. Neurasthenia.
254. Obesity.
255. Obesity.
256. Normal.
257. Chronic constipation.
258. Lumbago.

259. Obesity. Coronary sclerosis.
260. Cardiac neurosis.
261. Myalgia.
262. Normal.
263. Arterial hypertension.
264. Neurasthenia.
265. Myalgia.
266. Internal cranial hyperostosis.
267. Normal.
268. Cardiac neurosis.
269. Cardiac neurosis.
270. Hysteria.
271. Myalgia.
272. Cardiac neurosis.
273. Obesity.
274. Normal.
275. Coronary sclerosis.
276. Cholelithiasis.
277. Normal.
278. Chronic colitis.
279. Normal.
280. Chronic constipation.
281. Brachial neuritis.
282. Eczema.
283. Obesity.
284. Normal.
285. Neurasthenia.
286. Normal.
287. Asthenia.
288. Cardiac neurosis.
289. Morgagni's disease.
290. Neurasthenia.
291. Obesity.
292. Obesity.
293. Obesity.
294. Normal.
295. Normal.
296. Obesity.
297. Coronary sclerosis.
298. Neurasthenia.
299. Myalgia.
300. Syphilis.
301. Obesity.
302. Obesity.
303. Obesity.
304. Chronic bursitis.
305. Normal.
306. Normal.
307. Obesity.
308. Coronary sclerosis.

CASE RECORD NUMBERS FOR THE HYPOMETABOLISM MATERIAL

1: 924/41. 2: 1003/41. 3: 332/42. 4; 1506/42. 5: 301/40. 6: 117/42. 7: 1597/42. 8: 10[illegible]8/40. 9; 1475/42. 10: 813/40. 11: 1213/40. 12: 1507/42. 13: 1100/41. 14: 768/41. 15: 1361/42. 16: 1378/41. 17: 451/42. 18: 976/40. 19: 248/40. 20: 343/42. 21: 586/41. 22: 113/41. 23: 935/40. 24: 285/40. 25: 380/42. 26: 338/41. 27: 597/41. 28: 48/41. 29: 590/42, 30: 967/40. 31: 729/41. 32: 1118/41. 33: 1385/41. 34: 236/41. 35: 1447/42. 36: 212/40. 37: 1007/40. 38: 672/42. 39: 852/41. 40: 1005/40. 41: 952/41. 42: 549/42. 43: 115/40. 44: 635/41. 45: 676/41. 46: 542/41. 47: 425/41. 48: 1403/41. 49: 968/41. 50: 37/41. 51: 389/40. 52: 462/41. 53: 299/41. 54: 1097/40. 55: 906/41. 56: 1329/41. 57: 534/41. 58: 831/41. 59: 1066/41. 60: 764/41. 61: 1281/41. 62: 935/41. 63: 1249/41. 64: 1563/41. 65: 528/41. 66: 495/40. 67: 386/41. 68: 1014/41, 69; 1289/41. 70: 859/40. 71: 299/40. 72: 680/40. 73: 1073/40. 74: 1221/41. 75: 373/42. 76: 268/41. 77: 81/40. 78; 17/41. 79: 342/42. 80: 1481/41. 81: 475/40. 82: 63/41. 83: 1189/41. 84; 1170/41. 85: 668/40. 86: 829/40. 87: 227/42. 88: 800/41. 89: 211/41. 90: 851/40. 91: 881/40. 92: 445/40. 93: 1318/41. 94: 713/41. 95: 138/40. 96: 1224/41. 97: 1060/41. 98: 152/40. 99: 1035/41. 100: 646/41. 101: 916/41. 102: 905/40. 103: 799/40. 104: 383/42. 105: 1661/42. 106: 704/40. 107: 893/41. 108: 648/42. 109: 145/40. 110: 1017/40. 111: 990/42. 112: 972/40. 113: 1051/42. 114: 657/40. 115: 425/40. 116: 1067/41. 117: 885/41. 118: 960/41. 119: 1161/41. 120: 988/42. 121: 1429/41. 122: 800/40. 123: 1098/42. 124: 1155/41. 125: 1009/40. 126: 245/42. 127: 1229/40. 128: 614/41. 129: 856/41. 130: 226/40. 131: 1188/40. 132: 678/41. 133: 951/41. 134: 455/40. 135: 551/42. 136: 286/41. 137: 525/42. 138: 1180/40. 139: 809/41. 140: 1098/40. 141: 670/41. 142: 1630/42. 143: 1014/40. 144: 335/41. 145: 1110/40. 146: 689/41. 147: 381/40. 148: 58/41. 149: 79/41. 150: 1196/40. 151: 286/40. 152: 1442/41. 153: 1489/42. 154: 303/41. 155: 806/40. 156: 992/41. 157: 717/41. 158: 395/40. 159: 1317/42. 160: 1038/40. 161: 82/41. 162: 1445/42. 163: 830/42. 164: 955/40. 165: 839/41. 166: 940/42. 167: 544/42. 168: 674/41. 169: 840/42. 170: 823/41. 171: 1132/40. 172: 85/41. 173: 565/42. 174: 1159/40. 175: 886/41. 176: 223/41. 177: 765/40. 178: 1522/42, 179: 1486/41. 180: 943/40. 181: 480/40. 182: 324/41. 183: 250/40. 184: 202/41. 185: 298/41. 186: 932/40, 187: 1430/41. 188: 622/42. 189: 1159/40. 190: 663/41. 191: 636/40. 192: 85/42. 193: 182/42. 194: 323/40. 195: 191/42. 196: 1490/41. 197: 89/42. 198: 901/42. 199: 129/42. 200: 1002/41. 201: [illegible]09/40. 202: 679/42. 203: 691/41. 204: 937/41. 205: 790/41. 206: 875/41. 207: 702/41. 208: 1068/40. 209: 497/41. 210: 774/41. 211: 1417/41. 212: 313/41. 213: 106/42. 214: 1116/41. 215: 1180/42. 216: 1103/41. 217: 784/40. 218: 302/41. 219: 524/41. 220: 1407/41. 221: 1484/41. 222: 952/40. 223: 1021/40. 224: 889/42. 225: 287/41. 226: 643/41. 227: 607/40. 228: 1209/40. 229: 57/41. 230: 433/41. 231: 448/41. 232: 543/42. 233: 1013/40. 234: 351/42. 235: 230/41. 236: 754/41. 237: 1147/40. 238: 1246/41. 239: 1044/40. 240: 1209/41. 241: 975/41. 242: 1121/42. 243: 625/40. 244: 229/41. 245: 957/40. 246: 1040/40. 247: 532/41. 248: 1095/41. 249: 518/41. 250: 1073/41. 251: 1476/42. 252: 1353/41. 253: 961/41. 254: 354/41. 255: 100/41. 256: 380/41. 257: 1195/40. 258: 584/41. 259: 115/40. 260: 440/41. 261: 418/40. 262: 1257/41. 263: 826/40. 264: 989/40. 265: 866/42. 266: 1508/42. 267: 190/42. 268: 20/42. 269: 1293/41. 270: 472/40. 271: 865/42. 272: 675/40. 273: 655/40. 274: 1137/40. 275: 171/42. 276: 687/42. 277: 792/41. 278: 1189/40. 279: 539/42. 280: 238/41. 281: 480/41. 282: 442/41. 283: 519/40. 284: 1387/42. 285: 488/41. 286: 854/41. 287: 939/40. 288: 328/42. 289: 225/41. 290: 1472/42. 291: 881/41. 292: 1104/40. 293: 167/41. 294: 1220/42. 295: 896/41. 296: 837/41. 297: 474/40. 298: 325/41. 299: 1079/40. 300: 482/41. 301: 1151/40. 302: 688/41. 303: 771/42. 304: 1138/41. 305: 1041/41. 306; 130/41. 307: 445/41. 308: 911/42.

CLINICAL DIAGNOSES AND CASE HISTORY NUMBERS FOR PATIENTS IN THE CONTROL GROUP

SURVEY OF DIAGNOSES FOR THE CONTROL GROUP

Diagnosis	Number
Arthritis	15
Lumbago	4
Achylic anemia	1
Pernicious anemia	1
Obesity	12
Simple goiter	3
Gastric anacidity	2
Chronic alcoholism	1
Chronic colitis	4
Gastritis	11
Constipation	7
Chronic alcoholism	1
Carbon monoxide poisoning	1
Alopecia	1
Pruritus	2
Eczema	1
Urticaria	1
Convalescence	4
Gonorrhoea	1
Tape worm	2
Syphilis	1
Tuberculosis of the spine	2
Arterial hypertension	3
Cardiac neurosis	1
Myocarditis	4
Coronary sclerosis	2
Valvular heart disease	3
Paroxysmal tachycardia	1
Cerebral hemorrhage	2
Cerebral arteriosclerosis	4
Chronic encephalitis	2
Neuritis	2
Nervous anorexia	1
Mental depression	1
Hysteria	7
Neurasthenia	20
Psychosis	4
Nephritis	2
Malignancy	1
Hypogonadism	35
Normal	16

CASE RECORD NUMBERS FOR THE CONTROL GROUP

(Numbers given in italics indicate patients with hypogonadism)

304/41. 307/41. *308/41.* 318/41. 322/41. 339/41, 340/41. 342/41. 348/41. 391/41. 398/41. 401/41. 403/41. 405/41. 409/41. 410/41. 414/41. 415/41. 417/41. 420/41. 428/41. *436/41.* 446/41. 451/41. *453/41.* 458/41. 459/41. 466/41. 470/41. 475/41. 492/41. 494/41. *522/41.* 533/41. 538/41. *546/41.* 564/41. 565/41. 570/41. 572/41. 573/41. *575/41.* 579/41. 581/41. 588/41. 599/41. 600/41. 604/41. 609/41. *613/41.* 617/41. 621/41. *634/41.* *658/41.* 662/41. *665/41.* 700/41. 707/41. 723/41. 730/41. 733/41. 748/41. 749/41. 769/41. *771/41.* 773/41. 782/41. 786/41. 791/41. 804/41. *811/41.* 815/41. 820/41. 822/41. 824/41. 829/41. 832/41. 833/41. *844/41.* 847/41. 849/41. *851/41.* *857/41.* 863/41. 870/41. *871/41.* 872/41. 873/41. 876/41. 877/41. 879/41. 883/41. 887/41. 907/41. 913/41. 914/41. 919/41. 921/41. 923/41. 925/41. 931/41. 944/41. 953/41. 963/41. 969/41. 976/41. *980/41.* 985/41. 986/41. 1004/41. 1007/41. 100941. 1012/41. 1017/41. 1022/41. 1023/41. *1040/41.* 1047/41. *1049/41.* 1055/41. 1072/41. 1074/41. 1087/41. 1104/41. *1105/41.* 1106/41. 1109/41. 1119/41. 1120/41. 1122/41. 1123/41. 1132/41. 1137/41. 1144/41. 1148/41. *1163/41.* 1172/41. 1174/41. 1176/41. 1181/41. 1186/41. 1187/41. 1204/41. 1206/41. 1221/41. *1232/41.* 1243/41. 1247/41. *1254/41.* 1255/41. 1259/41. 1271/41. 1272/41. 1276/41. 1283/41. 1292/41. 1317/41. 1323/41. 1346/41. 1352/41. 1357/41. 1371/41. 1372/41. 1373/41. 1374/41. 1380/41. 1390/41. 1397/41. *1405/41.* *1410/41.* *1435/41.* 1437/41. *1450/41.* *1456/41.* *1459/41.* *1467/41.* *1495/41.* 1539/41. *1541/41.* 1552/41. 1554/41. 2/42. 4/42. 8/42. 21/42. *30/42.* 47/42. 60/42. *71/42.* *90/42.*

Printed in Dunstable, United Kingdom

91221455R00051